scratching

the

surface

BATTLING ECZEMA, CONQUERING
TOPICAL STEROID WITHDRAWAL AND
FINDING HOPE IN THE CHAOS

ALLYSON STEEDMAN

First published by Calathea Press 2022

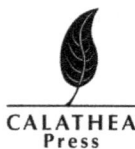

CALATHEA
Press

Cover design and interior typesetting by Laura Boyle Design

ISBN 978-1-7386652-0-4 (print)

ISBN 978-1-7386652-1-1 (ebook)

First edition

Carrying much symbolism across many cultures, the woodpecker is a mighty force. Associated with strength, courage, wisdom and kindness, its tenacity in life reminds us to continually persevere with a prevailing determination. It sees the opportunity in every situation and reminds us of all that can be found when we scratch the surface and unveil what lies beneath.

Table of Contents

Introduction

"You should be a writer—you have a way with words."
That's what my husband, Andrè, said to me this year. A
short time after, my mom echoed the sentiment. I had
loved to write when I was younger, but it was mostly
stop-and-start fictional stories and song lyrics. Stuff my
teenage self was emotionally drawn to. I always enjoyed
writing, even though I was never particularly good at it;
in fact, it was the one school subject that I struggled with
at times. Maybe it was the structured nature of writing
an opening theme, developmental middle, and conclusive
ending that challenged me. I was more free in my thinking, preferring to weave my story outside the confines of
curriculum. When I had to write because it was expected
of me, it was a chore—and a bore, really. When I wrote
for myself, it was exhilarating. My imagination wouldn't
cease: a torrent of ideas, thoughts, and stories was constantly flowing through my head. I would have hundreds
of creative bursts explode into story beginnings, only to
fizzle as I tried feebly to see an idea go further than its

beginning. So, while I enjoyed writing and had lots of creative ideas, actually writing something of value or meaning was not really an aspiration I entertained.

But on the day my husband told me I should write, a little spark ignited in my soul, like an ember trying to catch fire. It was without any wind or air yet to help it flame, but it was flickering nonetheless.

Perhaps it was the deep knowing I've had inside me for, really, my entire life: that I wanted and needed to connect through words. But I lacked the courage or honesty to step into a realm I had long ago told myself was an impossibility.

How do you make something happen when it seems impossible to do? How do you propel yourself into something that, on the surface, appears out of reach, is daunting to attempt, and might be completely out of left field?

Writing something for someone else to read, while always a dream at a subconscious level, was definitely an idea that I never before had the courage to manifest. The sharing of personal thoughts, ideas, and life experiences was reserved for those closest to me—and really, only my husband was privy to almost all my thoughts. I held lots of things close to my chest. We all do this to some degree, and it's important to know who you can tell certain things to and how much you can share. A measured distance in many of our relationships is healthy in order to protect ourselves from emotional vampires. But at the time I was very closed off, and I needed to learn to share my dreams and my insecurities. To vocalize my vulnerabilities and to embrace support and help from those whom I trusted.

It took time, but it is because of that openness that this writing came to fruition.

I do have to confess that I had a major life experience that helped to percolate this book. It changed me so dramatically that I felt this pull to share, in the hope that my story could help others to heal. When Andre kept telling me over and over that I was such a good writer, I really didn't believe him. Actually, he had been telling me this for years, but it wasn't until earlier this year, as I worked on reconnecting with my true soul and purpose, that I really did hear him. Or rather, listen to him. All those times before I was still the old Allyson, the uncertain, wavering woman who never fully embraced her own gifts. I was often embarrassed about my own thoughts, my own voice, that I wouldn't sound intellectual enough or educated enough or that my words and story would be meaningless to others.

This health journey I endured forced me to wake up and dig deep. It was a painful experience because, well, trying to better yourself often is. But it has given me so much drive to be open and share and, ultimately, heal for good.

My skin challenges were what directed me to this path right now, sharing my story and help with you. It was my sign, and like Andre had told me, I needed to write it all down. But let me be clear: I am not a doctor or a researcher. I am not a geneticist. I do not have a medical background, nor do I have a degree in writing or journalism. I don't pretend to have the answers. What I do have is my story, and it's a true story. All I can do is relay what happened to me and what I've come through. How my physical journey to heal led me down a spiritual path of rediscovering myself and making changes to support a healthy and healing life in the future. It is this story—my story—that I share with you.

I took the first step into the intimidating unknown territory of doing what frightens me. I am here with you now because I stopped listening to that voice that says no and started to believe in what someone else told me. I trusted in Andre's assessment of my abilities and I put down my shield and dove in. I needed to share my challenge and journey, and the pages that follow are me stepping out of the shadow and living in the light.

Chapter 1

BACK TO THE BEGINNING

This book is really twofold. It is about my physical journey, one that has spanned my entire life and led me down an unknown and treacherous path. And it is about how that journey led to an awakening, or rather a reawakening, of who I was and who I really wanted to be. In order to get to the end, I have to start at the beginning.

I am someone like everyone else. I live a life, have family and friends, and strive to find balance in all that I do. Like everyone else, I have issues and insecurities and struggles. I am not extraordinary or special or unique. I am just like everyone else. At least, that's what I told myself until I realized that no one is like anyone else.

But I'll get to that. For now, I have to start where it all began. With me, and the other part of me: my skin.

For my entire life, I have been two halves of a whole. I was born on June 7, 1976, a Gemini. And while I always took a secret pride in being the communicator sign of the zodiac and a chameleon able to function and move between different groups and topics with ease, I had no idea how my sign's duality would form much of the basis of me and everything I did. Not a good-and-bad duality, but two very different parts of a whole picture. An introvert at heart and social butterfly when needed, a confident-girl exterior and an anxiety-ridden interior, an excellent counsellor to others but a terrible advisor to myself. An exterior-me shown to the world as confident and in control, but an interior-me that always battled myself. Much of this duality I love, much of it I hate. It has been so ingrained in me that it has been difficult to separate the two, but this journey has helped me do that so much along the way. My skin solidified these two parts of me in ways I am only now able to measure.

My parents are great people. They married young after meeting at university. They wanted to start a family but found it very difficult. After many years of trying without success, my mom, a teacher, decided to pursue a master's degree while my dad focused on building his career in finance. It was time for them to move on and think about what a life and marriage would be without a biological child. Shortly after their decision to move in a new direction, my mom found out that she was pregnant. My parents were excited of course, but my mom's pregnancy wasn't an easy one: touch and go right from the beginning. She was very ill during the first trimester, spending time in the hospital because she was at risk to miscarry. She told me about interacting with her hospital roommate, who had miscarried and was actually quite happy about it. For a young woman who had been through so much already to have her own child, this other patient wasn't easing her mind. But my mom made it through the first trimester and was able to go back to work for a bit. She carried me full-term and I was born at a healthy weight of seven pounds, six ounces. While I know that my mom's pregnancy was a challenging time for her, both my parents told me that they were elated to finally welcome me into the world.

One of the most fortunate relationships in my early life was with our family doctor. He was kind, supportive, and understanding. Thorough and experienced, he noticed things. Soon after I was born, he detected a deformity in my hip socket. My leg had not fully formed into the socket and would need treatment; otherwise, I would walk with a limp and face other complications later in life. The "fix" was to wear an absurdly large diaper to compress the leg into the socket. A simple solution, except for a small problem that many would overlook. But the stage had already been set for my parents for a life of stress and anxiety where their daughter was concerned.

My skin became the other part of me when I was about six months old. I was diagnosed with eczema, a chronic inflammatory condition in which the skin develops a rash and cycles between oozing and weeping and being intensely dry and itchy. Much more common today, in the 1970s eczema was not regularly diagnosed and treating it was somewhat of an enigma. There is some truth in it being a hereditary condition: with both my parents experiencing skin issues when they were younger, it was inevitable that I would have some form of it as well. For two young parents, who had wanted a child for so long, to be faced with first a physical problem with their daughter's leg, and now with a chronic diagnosis of her incurable skin condition, I can only imagine the stress and sadness they must have felt. I always felt their love, always had their support, but it wasn't until I was a parent myself that I fully understood the amount of resolve needed to deal with my issues on a daily basis. Because it was bad, right from the beginning. That was when my skin became me and I became it. Every conversation and interaction would now involve equating my skin with who I was as a person.

My memory bank doesn't include the early stages, when I was too young to comprehend or understand what was really going on. I have the pictures though, and it's heartbreaking to look at a young baby and toddler with a swollen red face, hands covered with cracks and sores. While I didn't have the knowledge yet to be embarrassed or sad about my skin, my mom did. It was the most difficult on her. She was the primary caregiver, constantly faced with the maddening sounds of the daily itch and scratch. Unable to escape from the dry skin, rashes, and blood, along with facing all the challenges that come with navigating the first few years of a little life, she had little reprieve from the anxiety.

In those early years, our house didn't have air conditioning, so my mom would often take me out in the middle of those humid summer nights and drive us around in our air-conditioned car to find some cooling relief. Sleep was a series of fits and starts for me, and it was elusive for her. Life was filled with fatigue, worry, frustration and helplessness. People didn't really understand my condition and everywhere we went they would stare at me, at my swollen and oozing skin. Many times we couldn't hide the rashes or the bleeding, and my mom had to bolster herself against the stares and whispers from strangers. These reactions were probably more from confusion than from scorn, but to a new mother it must have been unbearable.

As I mentioned, eczema wasn't a common condition at the time and little was really known about the causes. We hadn't made the connection between the body, diet, and mind yet, so my parents were mainly advised to treat outbreaks with corticosteroid creams. We spent countless hours at dermatologist appointments, and my parents spent thousands of dollars on medication. Every visit to the doctor resulted in the same response: I had an incurable condition and we just needed to manage the outbreaks. There was nothing else to do except remove a few things from my diet and try to make me as comfortable as possible when the situation became bad. The steroid creams were a wonderful reprieve from the itch. We applied them diligently and liberally and while they didn't prevent a flare from happening, they did a fantastic job of soothing the itch and ache and providing a break from the constant scratch. I took oatmeal baths regularly; and whatever else my parents were told or thought could help, we tried. Anything to stop the constant sound of scratching and the daily visual reminder of my always-in-turmoil body.

My skin wasn't just reserved for the three of us. Soon, it became apparent that it would be the silent companion lurking in the shadows of everywhere I went. My whole family—my aunt, uncles, cousins, and grandparents—would be touched by my issues. Some of my cousins' first memories are of us jumping and hollering on my grandma's bed with her yelling from the other room: "Allyson, stop your scratching." My grandma would wrap my hands in cotton socks to stop the scratch and would pull my hands and yell at me when I would reflexively be unable to stop. Her no nonsense Polish approach was always out of love and concern, but I think she too was often exasperated by the constant scratching. Conversations would often involve questions about how I was doing and offers of new creams to try. There was so much concern and love, but at times I just wished to escape.

As I grew, my skin became less of a separate identity and more of just who I was. It became less obvious to us and my family as we melded into life living with a chronic condition. We just kept going and living with it, trying to mitigate times of discomfort as best we could.

But those who suffer from eczema, especially at a young age, have a compromised immune system to a degree, and other autoimmune responses and ailments tend to develop at some point. Around grade four, I developed asthma and seasonal allergies. Initially I was prescribed the rescue puffer Ventolin to use when an asthma attack came on. It didn't have any steroid in it, but a quick puff of it helped open the airways to the lungs and provided immediate relief to being unable to breathe. The allergies were usually seasonal, and something that I just muddled through when they were triggered. A few years into my asthma diagnosis, my doctor wanted to better manage the inflammation in my lungs rather than simply respond to an attack. I was prescribed an inhaled steroid called Beclaforte, which I took twice a day. The consistent stream of steroid being sent to the lungs would help keep the inflammation down and, it was hoped, prevent any serious asthma attack. I still kept my rescue puffer close at hand, though, ready for any attack that may come.

Despite this managed medication, the asthma proved to be just as time-consuming and worrisome as my eczema. An attack could come on quickly. I took two puffs of Ventolin before any exercise or sport, and I had to keep a diligent watch on my surroundings for anything that could trigger an attack. I had to avoid an exhaustive (and exhausting) list of foods, animals, and environments that could set my body into fight mode—sometimes it felt like I was allergic or reactive to everything.

To say that our lives were dictated and controlled by my skin issues would be an understatement. It permeated every conversation and every decision that my family or I made. In time, it became impossible to think of myself as separate from my condition; there was no Allyson without eczema. It was me, and I was it. It was almost as if my skin was the dominant personality in me, one that overshadowed the true me, always taking centre stage. It was the first thing I thought about when I woke up, it consumed how I went through my day, and it was the last thing I thought about before falling asleep.

It constantly poked at me; that drip, drip, drip of irritation. Even when I didn't have a full-blown flare and things were manageable, I would itch or rub out of habit or some sort of nervous tick. My daily routine consisted of moisturizer application, cortisone cream application, deciding on clothes that would hide any breakout, and constant, constant anxiety about how I looked and what others saw.

As I progressed through childhood, my skin was like the albatross I couldn't shake. Even when the eczema was milder and manageable, just the very thought of it tormented me. I was embarrassed and often felt small compared to everyone else. Clear skin was an enigma to me, and I often fantasized about being free and carefree in my body. I was envious of the bare arms and legs of my friends.

By this time, my eczema had become such a strong part of my personality that I didn't know how to function without it. I was a nervous kid and not one to stand out. Whether my shyness was something inherent in me I can't be sure, but I am sure that my skin and subsequent embarrassment about its condition definitely held me back. So many times I just wanted to shrink and not be seen. Much of the time I longed to just blend.

This wasn't something that just affected me. Through the years it didn't get any easier for my parents, especially my mom. With a determination that I couldn't fully understand until I had a child myself, my mom spent the majority of her time not only physically helping me but also expending so much emotional turmoil. The inability to help your child when you see them suffering is something that so many parents can understand. The mental stability needed to stay strong when all you want to do is collapse in tears is difficult to endure. It's only as an adult that I can now fully understand and appreciate the stress that my condition must have put on my parents.

Most of my early life was spent in some stage of un-well. Between my eczema flares (sometimes severe) and my asthma and allergies, something always needed tend-ing to. My immune system was constantly compromised, and I would fall ill at least once a year like clockwork. Strep throat was a given, and my body cycled through many rounds of antibiotics.

The frustrating part was that even through all the dermatologist and specialist appointments, all the time spent rearranging schedules and driving to various hospi-tals and clinics, no indication of any cure or a timeline for outgrowing or recovering from eczema was ever given. The diagnosis was always the same: this was a lifelong, chronic condition with no cure. We would have to learn to live with it and manage it as best we could.

So, we all accepted it. And life moved on.

This isn't to say that everything was all doom and gloom. In fact, it was quite the opposite. While my skin was something that just became a part of my narrative, my life as a whole was really wonderful. Despite my health issues, I had a tremendous upbringing. My dad was a business exec-utive and my mom was a teacher, and together they worked hard to improve our lifestyle, instilling a strong work ethic in me. My parents were very supportive, kind, and giving. They enjoyed theatre, music, museums, architecture, and travel. I learned to appreciate the value of a good book from my dad and how to compose myself with elegance and grace from my mom. We travelled quite a bit, and I was exposed to so much culture and other countries that it sparked and fuelled a passion for discovery and travel that I still carry throughout my life. And while we didn't sit down for life discussions or say I love you at all, I had a knowing in my heart that they were the two people in my life who loved me unconditionally. While we weren't a family of words, we were a family of action, and both my parents spent time with me and gave me the attention that helped me feel safe and cared for at all times. We were close and home always felt like a safe haven for me, a place where I could escape the world and just be me. The most important lesson I learned from my parents, though, was perseverance. They encouraged me to keep going and at no point did they allow me to wallow in self-pity or give up because of my skin. They taught me, simply through their actions, that we all come up against obstacles in our life, whether they be temporary or long-term, and it is how we push through that is the characteristic that we should nurture.

I didn't realize it at the time, but the duality of my life was merging with most of my existence. I was living two ways: happy, excited, and optimistic about what the future held; and uncertain, worried, and concerned with how I was perceived and accepted. I had the passion, dedication, and determination of my parents that fuelled the action needed to set goals and strive to achieve them, but this was coupled with my internal struggle to be normal, and to be the same as everyone else, at least from a physical perspective.

It's interesting to look back through the lens of time and see myself objectively. I didn't realize then that my skin condition had a real impact on my personality and the way I interacted with others. I can see now that my constant embarrassment and humiliation encouraged more shyness and uncertainty. How the eczema triggered in me a longing to belong and to not be judged. To be valued for who I was as a person, not for what was seen on the outside. I wanted a different narrative than the kid with terrible skin. It was this early years moulding that I would carry throughout my life.

I guess that's why I held hard to doing well in school and being perfect in what I did. I wanted more out of life and I didn't want my skin to hold me back. If I was poised and thoughtful, hardworking and conscientious, then I would be liked, or admired, and have something more to give than my physical appearance. I was determined to do well in school, to make my parents proud and give them something more exciting to talk about when the topic turned to me. Unknowingly, I strived to do what they thought was right, or acceptable, because I had already caused so much upheaval and pain. I wanted them to be proud of me and what I achieved, and I just wanted to do well and not be a further problem.

As I grew and settled into adolescents, my skin became much easier to manage. I still had outbreaks, but they were usually because of lack of sleep or stress from schoolwork. My asthma continued to be a real issue, but finally I was starting to feel more comfortable in my own skin and connected to who I really was. The fears and uncertainties were still there, but I didn't feel handcuffed to my skin condition anymore. I was able to live with my skin, doing daily maintenance to try to keep any flares at bay. I had a sense of security that, while I would have to live with this condition forever, it wouldn't control me anymore or dictate how I lived. It would always be a part of me, but I didn't feel defined by it. More importantly, I didn't live in constant fear and worry that my skin *might* get out of control.

I continued along in my high school years with pretty much normal skin. I had a few bumps along the way: an outbreak one summer when I spent too much time in the sun, and many bouts of strep throat if I wasn't taking great care of myself. I started to feel pretty too. For most of my young childhood, I didn't feel any way about how I looked other than embarrassed, but as I got older and had longer stretches of good, manageable skin, especially on my face, I leaned in a bit to feeling attractive and like everyone else. If I did have an outbreak, it was much easier to hide in those years and I could focus on my hair, makeup, and clothes. I felt like a normal teenager, concerned about grades and boys and finding that I didn't need to give much attention to my skin. What was part of me no longer defined me.

That sense of security and optimism changed quickly, however, in my last year of high school. It wasn't until I was eighteen years old, in a foreign country, living away from my parents, that I would first experience an issue with my skin that was more than just an annoyance or an embarrassment. It was the first time in my life that I was scared, really scared, about what could happen to my body and what my body could become.

Chapter 2

VIVE LA FRANCE

My parents worked very hard on their careers. Sometime in the early to mid-1980s, my dad's career progressed onto a huge trajectory. While initially starting his career as an accountant, my dad would proceed to hold advancing positions in the finance department of various companies, and after completing his MBA, jumped into the executive suite. Soon, he was Executive Vice President for an international printing and packaging company whose work took him to all parts of the globe. His company had a head office in Toronto, with a secondary European office in London and it was there that he would spend a lot of his time. For about ten days to two weeks every month or so, my dad would be working abroad, headquartered in London. My mom and I spent a lot of time together. We'd miss him when he was gone, but we soon settled into a routine that became normal for us. This was before cellphones and email, a time when the only way to communicate was calling through a land line or actually posting a letter. We would hope to hear from him, but it was often difficult to coordinate the best time to connect, given the time difference. When the phone rang, we would go running to answer.

Despite missing him when he was away, his job did provide some amazing perks for us and I got to experience so much at such a young age: not only memories that shaped me but also ones that I will cherish forever. Every summer we would travel to London together; and throughout the year, if we were able to manage with my school and my mom's teaching position, we would accompany my dad on trips to other places in the world. The year I was thirteen provided the most experiences for us. My mom took the year off to regroup and accompany my dad on some of his business trips. Even though I was in school and couldn't go with them all the time, I got to join them on some amazing trips during my March and Summer breaks from school. We travelled to Hawaii and Japan, England and France. London held my heart, but it was Paris that held my imagination. The romance, the culture, and the wonderful way the French had of slowing life down, enjoying the moment and really living, captured my longing. It was such the antithesis to the often frantic, fast-paced North American culture that I could easily get lost in my fantasies about it.

We toured the Louvre, found our favourite shops for pain au chocolat, had lunch atop the Eiffel Tower, and strolled along the Seine. It was spring in Paris: I still don't think anything can compare.

After we came home, I didn't know when I would see Paris again, or when I would even visit France again. This was a once-in-a-lifetime trip, since I didn't see it happening again any time soon. I savoured the pictures and images in my mind and imagined a time when I would be there again. It was fantasy, I knew, but I felt a connection to the city, the country, and the people. I had no way of knowing at the time that five years later I would not only be visiting France again but living there.

I've always had a wanderlust about me. My spirit and my soul felt intoxicated with the smells and sounds of other cities. I loved to explore and—whether fuelled by my earlier exposure to travel or something that just felt right to me—I longed to always get away and be somewhere unknown. Our stays in London each year solidified my connection to Europe. I felt at home and at ease, even in bustling and populated cities. While my home in Canada was always my home, the world intrigued and enticed me. I forever longed to be somewhere else and to experience something new.

So it was surprising to me when one day I ran across an advertisement in the newspaper for a Canadian school abroad. I had just been skimming, looking for some entertainment news, and there, right in front of me in bold type, were details for an information night about the Lycée Canadien en France. I didn't really think much about it at first, didn't register any details. But the thought lingered, and I couldn't shake thinking about what this place was and what it meant. I was interested and intrigued and when I showed my parents the advertisement, they too had an interest to learn more. We went to the information night without any expectations, but when I left I was filled with excitement. It sounded too amazing, too right for me. Nervously, I approached my parents to discuss whether this could even be an option for me. It didn't scare me to be away from home, I didn't feel any anxiety, only a desire to make it happen. My wanderlust had ignited.

My parents were people of action and while I know that my mom was a ball of worry, they both loved to travel and knew the experience I would get could never be replicated. I had already done a lot of travelling, so that wasn't a concern, and I understood some French. Together, we decided that this was a journey I had to take.

The year leading up to leaving was a flurry of excitement. While I was finishing up grade twelve, I also navigated choosing classes, organizing clothes, registering for a student visa, figuring out calling cards; the list went on and the year passed quickly. I felt great. Optimistic. A bit apprehensive but excited for this next chapter in my life. My skin was amazing too. Everything seemed to be going in the right direction.

By some twist of fate, one of my mom's good friend had called to say that the daughter of one of her friends was going to Lycée at the same time as me. She would love to get us all together for lunch so we could meet and, at the very least, know a familiar face when both of us arrived in France. I was really looking forward to meeting Stacey and her mom. Even if we didn't totally mesh, it would be amazing to actually know someone else who would be attending the school and see a familiar face when it was time to leave. The four of us met one summer afternoon in Toronto, and our lunch couldn't have gone any better. I liked Stacey from the first moment we met, and our moms got along too. Conversation flowed easily and we found that we had a lot in common. Nothing was awkward. It felt like this was finally really happening. I knew Stacey and I would be fast friends, and any trepidation I had was whisked away by utter enthusiasm.

The rest of the summer passed quickly. I worked full-time and spent as much of my free time with my friends before I was to leave. About a week before departure, the school sent us our schedules and rooming information. I had opted to stay with a French family instead of in residence because I felt that it would be more immersive for me and help provide the full experience of life there. By another amazing twist of fate, without either of us making the request, Stacey and I were placed together as roommates. We couldn't believe that everything was falling into place so well. And even though I didn't realize it at the time, it was an early indication and reminder that the Universe will always have my back I would see the same pattern throughout my life of people or situations coming and going that seem like coincidences or luck but are actually fatefully orchestrated.

Finally, September arrived and it was time to depart. I had all my bags packed and had included my asthma inhalers and steroid cream. I wasn't bringing a lot of cream because my eczema had been so great for so long. It was an afterthought, just in case. I had reached a point in my life where I felt that eczema was far behind me. Something that I could mark in my history and watch it through the rear-view lens. It was now something that my body would use to alert me if I wasn't taking care of it, or if it needed rest. A signal to do a bit better, rather than a mainstay in my everyday life. My separation from the condition was growing more in the divide, and I was feeling like I was able to detach my existence from my skin and really feel like I was able to be me.

The journey to France was arduous and long. We travelled as a large group, with administration from the school as our guide and chaperone, and it was pretty disorganized from the get-go. With a lengthy delay in Toronto, miscommunications, multiple layovers, and almost missed connections, it took more than twenty-four hours for us to arrive in Nice. We were tired, but we were here.

Our French mother picked us up from the airport and we communicated through various hand gestures and nervous laughs as our level of French was minimal and her understanding of English was non-existent. We packed into the car, felt the warmth of the Mediterranean sun through the window, and set off. Our home was in the seaside village of Villefranche-sur-Mer, a cozy town between Nice and Monaco. Our French mom stayed home with her three children and our French dad worked at the casino in Monte Carlo. The language barrier was tricky at times, but initially the family was welcoming and curious about these two young girls from Canada.

This area of the Mediterranean is built into corniches along the coast. Houses and apartments are built up along the hillside, and the topography has winding roads through the hills. Our home was situated up a steep hill from the road. While not large in its footprint, it rose four storeys from the street. Our room was on the first, or ground, floor. There was a main staircase that took visitors from the street up to the second level of the house, where the family lived. Our room was accessed from around the corner of the bottom of that staircase and had a small private entrance. It was a tiny room with ceilings not much higher than five feet or so. Stacey and I each had a twin bed with a table for studying down the middle of the room, separating our beds into our own little domains. There was a small windowless washroom and a little TV in the corner. Despite lacking some of the creature comforts that we had back home, it was our own private sanctuary and meant that we could have some quiet time away from the young family to attend to our schoolwork.

Despite my initial homesickness, Stacey and I settled into our space and soon became close friends. The first few weeks we navigated our way through new friendships, French train travel, and narrow streets. The weather was hot and our long walks along the Corniche left us and our friends drenched and drained. With our school, we went to some local cultural spots, tourist attractions, and lovely gardens. It was all so beautiful and so surreal, like nothing I had ever experienced before. The people, the water, the visuals were an assault on my senses but in the very best of ways.

The first month passed quickly. As October approached, my dad wrote to say that he would be coming to spend a week there to visit and explore with me. I was so happy. I was really enjoying myself and learning so much, but to have my dad there gave me a level of comfort and a feeling of home and I couldn't wait to see him. The weather was perfect when he arrived and he checked himself into a little pension in the town of St-Jean-Cap-Ferrat, just a short walk from my school. It wasn't a fancy place to stay, but it was comfortable and each morning he would have his continental breakfast on the balcony, meander the streets enjoying the culture and warmth, and then we would meet after school to explore. We'd have dinners in Villefranche, visit medieval cities like Eze, and drive around to explore everything together. It only enriched my experience so much more to have that time with him and create those memories. I felt lucky that he was able to come and join me and so grateful that I was having this experience at all.

So far it had been an amazing two months of living and learning. I was excited about and looking forward to what lay ahead. As I said goodbye to my dad until the Christmas holidays, I found myself energized about the remainder of the semester and keen on taking full advantage of everything the Côte d'Azur had to offer. I had no idea just how drastically my life would change in the months that followed and no idea of what I would be up against.

Chapter 3

A STORM IS BREWING

If the first two months of school sailed through on warm Mediterranean vibes, October through to December would prove to be much more challenging. Once the heatwave broke and October passed by, the rains started. Torrential rains. For days.

The rains were very challenging for Stacey and I. Our room was small and somewhat subterranean, so it quickly became damp and cold. We didn't have any heating available in our room and the one window at the front did not close properly. My bed covers would often feel wet from the moisture, and it was almost impossible for us to rid the room of the musky feel and dank texture. Gradually, black mould began to grow on the wall by the window and our towels would never really dry after our showers. The damp permeated everything in our room; even the pages of my textbooks would curl from the moisture.

While this was a nuisance and somewhat irritating for Stacey, it was a recipe for disaster for me. My skin issues started to rear up in ugly ways and very quickly got out of control. My skin had trouble breathing, and everything I did seemed to exacerbate the situation. Before I knew it, I was in a full-blown attack.

I attributed my outbreak to the dampness and mould in our room, but there was another factor that played into my skin's demise. I had run out of the limited supply of steroid cream that I used to keep my skin in check. I had no way of mitigating the attack. By December, my skin was so inflamed I wasn't able to turn my head. From my neck through my upper body and torso, I was ravaged by swollen, red, oozing skin. I didn't know what to do. I was so scared. I only worsened the situation by wearing clothing that tried to cover every inch of my body. While turtlenecks and hooded jackets concealed my burning skin, the heat caused my eczema to only burn more.

Stacey was my rock, always supportive and helpful, but likely scared and unsure herself. We were so close now, really great friends, but we had only known each other for a few months. She didn't know my history with eczema, and hadn't experienced one of my outbreaks or flares before. She must have been so scared yet kept it together for me. She was brave, and a true friend.

In hindsight, I think I was so frightened that I became immobile to my condition. Weeks went by and my skin only continued to spiral, yet I didn't do anything about it. Unsure of how to navigate the health system in France, and with a significant language barrier, I opted to tough it out and see my own doctor when I got home on Christmas break just a few weeks away.

The flight home couldn't go fast enough for me. Confined to my seat, out of necessity but mostly embarrassment, I watched movies on a constant stream during the eight-hour journey. I couldn't move my body and every attempted turn of my neck only elicited pain and increased discomfort. I just wanted to be home, to be safe and to crawl into my own bed and cry and cry. I have never been so grateful to land and to be home in my life.

As was the case upon arriving in France, my luggage was lost on the return to Toronto. Stacey went out a few minutes before me to find our parents while I made a claim about my things. I had been so oblivious to everything around me for so many weeks that I didn't realize that others saw what was happening to me. Stacey had never wavered in her friendship to me, never made mention of my skin, she just carried on. Her sensitivity extended even further when she left the arrivals lounge early to warn my parents about my appearance and to caution them not to let on how horrendous I looked. Her friendship and kindness were such a gift.

When I finally emerged from arrivals, I was overwhelmed at being able to see my parents and be in my own bed that night. It was evening as we drove home, and as the lights reflected off my window and the snow fell, I started to cry. The first real cry in all those weeks of suffering and uncertainty. A cry because now I was safe, at home with my parents, who would take care of me.

My mom was so distressed to see me in such discomfort and pain that she called our doctor, who agreed to see us after hours. Exhausted from the long travels home, weeks of torment from my skin, and coupled with my high emotions, I was a delirious mess. I only remember driving there in tears, desperate for some reprieve. The time in the doctor's office and the rushing to the pharmacy was all a blur to me. Our doctor prescribed a heavy dose of antibiotics and additional steroid cream and I was told to rest for a few days.

I spent much of my time home in hibernation, my mom fielding calls from my friends, and only going out for short periods of time. I slept almost straight through the first three days, my body trying desperately to heal. The rest, medication, and creams finally started working, and within about week I had rebounded and felt much better. I still had sores, scabs, and scars, but the burning feeling and fire-red skin had thankfully subsided.

Christmas came and I felt much better and cheerful. As New Year's passed and the time for me to return to school approached, I felt like my old self again. The memory, though, of how quickly my skin could deteriorate and the length to which my body could betray me never dimmed; and while I continued to move forward, I could never forget.

The rest of the year at school transpired really well. Stacey and I returned to our family and we had planned to finish our year living there. After a few days, it was clear that remaining in the home wouldn't be possible for us. They had cleaned up as best they could when we were away, but the mould was not removed, simply painted over, and the musky and damp feeling remained. My asthma started to act up, and we knew that to stay there would mean severe issues for my skin again. We decided it was best to move into the school residence until the end of the year. My skin was never a problem again and I was sure to have a stocked supply of steroid cream in case of emergency. My parents joined me for graduation, and we spent one last final week in the Mediterranean paradise.

Looking back with my future lens, I realize that I was experiencing the first stages of withdrawal but just didn't know it. How ironic that more than twenty years later I would be in the same position again, this time of my own choosing. The Universe was trying to alert me to something back then, but I didn't have the resolve, time, or understanding to heed the call then. I'm not sure I had the resolve or courage to answer it some twenty years later either, but I did—and that is the second part of my journey.

Chapter 4

THE NEXT CHAPTER

Throughout most of my time in France, I obsessed about getting into university, more specifically, my preferred university. I felt immense pressure to carry on in post-secondary education, partly from the expectations of my parents but mostly from myself. I had been given every advantage to succeed, and whether actually true or not, I felt that other people would deem me a failure if I didn't use those advantages to continue on. It was a running joke among my friends at school that I would constantly obsess and fret about not getting into my chosen school.

Needless to say, I got in. And I was thrilled. I had everything planned out; I would do two years undergraduate with a business focus, apply to attend the business school, and complete two years with an honours in business from the prestigious business school on campus. While the competition to get into the "biz school" was fierce, there was no doubt in my mind that I would attend.

My first couple of years at school were fantastic. The year I had spent in France had allowed me the space to mature and grow, which, although I hadn't realized at the time, really helped me to acclimatize to university life quite quickly. I was blessed too, with no skin issues. Finally, I had reached a point in my life where my decisions and movements were not dictated by my skin. I was free, to be me. My episode in France a distant memory. Even though it was something that I had vowed I would never forget, I fell into the patterns of life again and pushed that unhappy time to the back of my mind.

I enjoyed the freedom of school, the academics, campus life. I made friends, socialized, joined a sorority, lived. It was wonderful.

By my second year, I had to think about my application to the business school. My undergraduate degree was more rigorous than others—a higher grade-point average had to be maintained to remain in the program—and I thought this might work to my advantage when applying to the HBA program. I wasn't the top student in my class, but I had other things on my résumé that rounded out my application: international travel, studied and lived abroad, member of a sorority, and involved in many campus activities. The one prerequisite course was Biz 257, which wasn't my favourite class and I didn't always participate as much as I probably should have. To be honest, I found it boring and not totally up my alley, but it was what I needed to take if I wanted to get into the business school. The most important component of the class was the feasibility study. This group project culminated with a presentation of our idea and was the biggest undertaking of mine at university. It was an all-consuming project that had long been echoed throughout the halls as something that would take over your life for a bit. My group of seven brainstormed ideas and finally settled on the concept of a bar that sold specialty beers, made by a local brewery. It was daring, to say the least. At a time when products and corporate ideas were the mainstay in the class, conceptualizing a service idea, and a high-end bar nonetheless, was never heard of, let alone entertained.

We poured ourselves into the project, snagging any spare moment and pulling long hours to get everything done. While the project on paper was good, it was our presentation that really shone. Each group was to present in front of their class and each classmate was to vote on which presentation was the best, but you couldn't vote on your own. Ultimately, we won. We progressed to the semi-finals and then we were one of three groups who presented in the finals. We gave it our all, and although we didn't win, at least two of the judges approached us afterwards to congratulate us on our presentation style, with one even offering to hear more if we actually went through with our business. Naturally with all that fanfare, I figured I had a "biz school" acceptance in the bag.

Four of my team members were accepted. I was not.

I realize now that everything really does happen for a reason, but at the time, my whole focus, the main reason I even wanted to attend this particular university, had been shattered, throwing me off balance. I needed to pivot, and quickly. It was fortunate that I was currently enrolled in a business program so, while I wouldn't be armed with an HBA, I did have a great degree upon graduation. And I knew I wanted to pursue something in business like my dad, but I didn't know what. The focused approach of the business school was possibly too limiting for me, and staying the course in my current degree would prove to support me better. At least I would have more time on my hands; the HBA's notorious workload meant students didn't have much time for anything else.

And really, it was a blessing in disguise. Two of my third-year roommates and friends were in the HBA program. They loved it, but I didn't find it exciting. I was enjoying smaller class sizes, thought-provoking debates, and a freedom from the books that my current degree provided. I helped to produce and choreograph a fashion show on campus as well as participate in another one benefiting the city museum. And I was able to do a lot of things with my sorority. If I had attended the program, I likely wouldn't have met my husband or, at the very least, have had the time to really get to know him as a friend. Disappointments and setbacks are only temporary, and quite often the alternative is better in the end. It was another example of how the Universe was there for me, steering me in the direction that was better suited for me, helping me along the way, even when I didn't understand or realize it while it was happening.

What was most interesting during this time was how my skin performed. Needless to say, the excessive stress about getting into the business school would have caused my skin to flare. The late nights, lack of sleep, and general poorer nutrition would historically have pushed my immune system over the edge and triggered an outbreak. While I did have small recurrences of eczema, I would immediately apply steroid cream directly to the site and any additional flare would be contained. I didn't have to worry that it would develop into a full-blown attack and I felt secure in knowing that any minor outbreak could easily be cleared up by a little cream.

I finished out my final year and looked forward to what was next. I looked for work and spent many weekends going for interviews or revising my résumé. I had promising options, but nothing materialized into more. I pounded the pavement, and it was a tough go. I decided that I likely would have to continue on with school to make my background more robust. My next pivot was to take a Public Relations Post Graduate Certificate.

After my last day of classes, I packed my room, said goodbye to campus life, and went back to live with my parents for the year.

Throughout my whole time at university, I barely thought about my skin. In fact, it wasn't really a part of me anymore. The feeling of being free from my condition allowed me to really come out of my shell and thrive at just being me. I had never before met so many people whom I had fun with, or even connected with. I didn't have my skin holding me back, so I wasn't afraid to go out, flirt, laugh, socialize. It was an amazing feeling to be so carefree, so unencumbered.

My year at home actually went really well too. After being so independent for more than four years, I worried about how my parents and I would navigate around having my freedom while respecting that I was living under their roof. My schooling took up a lot of my time with driving there and back, sometimes eating up hours on the highway. If I wasn't working at my part-time job, I was home throughout the week doing hours of schoolwork and finishing projects, seeing friends, and staying over in the city on the weekends.

I was also finding more of my groove with what I liked to pursue. I had first chosen to attend university to pursue some offshoot of the business world. I did this mostly because my dad had been so successful and I wanted to find that as well. Also partly because I thought it would make my parents proud of me. With a powerful job that sounded important, I thought I would meet my earlier belief that I had to make something of all the advantages I was given. I didn't give much thought to what actually excited me or fired me up; I just wanted to do something that my parents could brag about. Throughout the coursework of my Public Relations diploma, however, I was finding that PR was definitely more suited to my personality. Not only did it allow me access to the business world I wanted to be a part of, but there were so many aspects of PR where I could use more of my creativity.

The year at college went quickly and I found myself in the same position as I did the year before: looking for a job. I sent out hundreds and hundreds of inquiries. It was 1999, a time when you still mailed in your résumé and called to follow up. I rarely, if ever, used email because most employers preferred fax and snail mail. The Internet was still new, and I would have to wait for what felt like hours while my computer waited for the dial-up connection to confirm I was online. Often I would be sending résumés blindly, not knowing if the companies I was contacting had any openings at all in the area I wanted to pursue.

Eventually, after a few months, I landed a few interviews, but so far the fit hadn't been right. But one last interview, at a company downtown, turned out to be great and afterwards I was offered the job. I was hired to be a marketing assistant in the Event Planning Department.

I started working in September 1999, and for the first few months I commuted from my parents' home. Over the course of the fall, we looked for a place for me to live downtown and soon found the perfect condo for me to move into. During this time, I reconnected with and started spending time with my friend Andre from university. Serendipitously, we worked right across the street from each other and our previous friendship at university lent a certain ease to us getting to know each other further without all the social distractions of school. We started dating and within a few years we were engaged and married, leaving downtown to start our life together in the suburbs of Toronto.

Life was moving on, and I was more excited than ever about what the future would hold.

Chapter 5

CAN'T SEEM TO ESCAPE IT

The eyes of retrospect are frustratingly clear. As I look back now, I can see how I continued to function with a level of held beliefs that permeated everything I did. My skin had been fairly consistent throughout my late teens and early twenties, yet the coping mechanisms and personality traits that I'd developed because of my feelings toward my skin at a young age carried through and were now the voices that second-guessed much of what I did. The duality was still there, although masked for some years.

Sure, my job, my wedding, and my relationship were seemingly moving along like they all should, but the pervasive need to be perfect clung to all that I touched. My desire to be liked and not rock the boat found its way into my career, and often I felt that my ideas, thoughts and opinions were hijacked by conformity if they deviated from the norm. I didn't want to create issues, or be reprimanded, or, heaven forbid, be fired, so I allowed my uncertainty to manifest into compliance. Soon, I felt lost in my job, tethered to the stability of work but feeling unfulfilled and challenged in my everyday duties. The tension I felt with a coworker who was first my boss and then my peer was a difficult obstacle to navigate, and I felt myself stressed and anxious as each day, month, and year progressed. My skin wasn't what was affecting me now, but the thoughts I spoke to myself and the anxieties I had created so far in my past were constantly present.

That's how we're all the same, really. For me, it was my skin; for others, it was their weight, or neglect, or some other trauma or experience at such a young age that defined who we were and are. Yes, we are the same as everyone else, but no one is really the same as anyone else.

Of course, I see that now, after everything, but it wasn't obvious to me then. Or rather, I wasn't obvious to it. Things are always clear if we're ready to see them. What needed to change wasn't what had been hidden in the shadows: it was my willingness to bring them to light.

Chapter 6

LIFE GETS CONFUSING

One thing that I didn't really worry about much was my skin. Stressful situations at work, my wedding, buying our first home: none of these caused any disruption to my skin. In the past, events like these would have definitely caused major outbreaks. I had small flares of eczema, but nothing that wasn't manageable. In fact, for all the time Andre had known me, he had only seen me experience mild skin issues. It was like an ancient past that I had no interest or desire to uncover again. I was free, functioning like everyone else, without constraint. I almost forgot that I had ever suffered at all.

A few years after Andre and I got married, we welcomed our daughter, Sydney. The first year was a flurry of activity and learning, laughter and tears, and lots and lots of worry. She was so inquisitive, even in that first year, and she constantly kept Andre and I engaged and on pointe. Combined with all the first-time-parent worries like checking if she was still breathing in the night, it was a very active year for us. I didn't realize it at the time, but my skin was the best it had ever been. It was radiant. Maybe it was the hormones or my age (I was thirty), but I probably hadn't looked or felt better in my life. I can only say this now as I look back on pictures of the time. In my reality then, I took for granted that I had great skin. I didn't appreciate it or give it any thought. I was too caught up in all the new mom stuff and my changing world that I didn't give any credit to my body.

When Sydney was about three years old, things started to change. As someone who had been relatively healthy for the past ten years or so, I started experiencing some strange and at times worrisome health issues. At first it was my voice. I would lose it. For days. At the time, I was pursuing creative outlets like singing lessons and some non-union acting gigs. It was something fun to do for myself, but I thought that maybe the overuse of my voice was causing the issue. So I cut back on my lessons and passed on some auditions as a way to rest my voice. Things improved, but ultimately I found myself struggling again.

This back-and-forth went on for about three years. I was referred to an ear, nose, and throat doctor, who concluded that nothing was wrong, but my voice would still leave me for no apparent reason. When this cycle kept continuing, I took a weekend course offered at the Stratford Festival, a Shakespearean repertory theatre company. I learned the Alexander Technique, a way of breathing and speaking that helps actors when they lose their voices. Still, no permanent change. I finally sought out a speech pathologist, and through various voice exercises I tried to retrain my vocal abilities. After about five weeks, my voice decided to stay and I never lost it again. Just as mysteriously as this issue had developed, it resolved with no real understanding of the cause or cure.

About a year or so later, I developed migraine headaches, many times catching me off guard. I had never experienced them before and it was very unsettling. I now understood why those who suffered from them needed to spend time in the dark, lying down, with no stimulus. For an entire summer I would have migraine attacks that would leave me alone in my bedroom for hours, altering weekend plans with my family and leaving me exhausted. My doctor's only solution was to prescribe medication that I would need to take the minute I felt a migraine coming on. Sometimes it was difficult for me to anticipate an onset so I rarely, if ever, was able to use the medication. I stumbled through this new condition, but then, as with my voice, poof: the migraines disappeared.

Underlying all these strange developments was an irregular menstrual cycle, something that was out of the ordinary for me. I sought answers from my family doctor and had ultrasounds with no worrying results. My doctor didn't seem too concerned because I had no intention of becoming pregnant again. Sure, it was great not to stress about my period for a few months at a time, but that convenience was always met many months later with an extreme cycle lasting six or seven weeks at a time. As with the other two issues, all my doctor visits and examinations found nothing. It was pretty disconcerting because, while I wasn't in pain, my body was clearly not functioning in the way it should. Something was wrong, but I just couldn't nail it down.

When Sydney was around eight, my throat started having issues again. I developed some severe pain and it became difficult to swallow. It came on rather fast, so I went to my walk-in clinic. Given that strep throat was a constant for me when I was a child, I thought maybe it was gearing up to be a version of that again. The swab came back negative for strep, but the doctor told me that I had an abscess on the left side of my throat. I was prescribed an antibiotic and given a cortisone injection to reduce the swelling. If I didn't see an improvement within twenty-four hours, I was told to make my way to the hospital.

I didn't see any improvement; in fact, the pain only increased, sending my discomfort through the roof. After another visit to the walk-in clinic, I was referred to the emergency room and then again to another ear, nose, and throat specialist. My mom raced me there, and the doctor drained the abscess. I felt relief within hours. But why did it happen?

I couldn't connect the dots as to the reason I was experiencing all these issues and symptoms. Yes, my life (and body) had changed after having Sydney, but other than using a daily steroid puffer to control my asthma, and some topical steroid cream for my eczema when needed, I didn't use any medications. And my routines, eating habits, and exercise remained constant. I didn't have much added or unusual stress in my life. Why now, and what could be causing all my weird conditions?

During all these strange occurrences, I started to notice a re-emergence of my eczema. Nothing terrible, just some irritation on my hands and feet. I continued to apply my cortisone steroid creams and that helped to keep it at bay for a while. Until one day it didn't.

My eczema returned with a vengeance to my hands and feet. It was easier to control on my feet because they weren't as exposed to different elements, but my hands proved trickier as they were constantly coming into contact with soap and water. The eczema was now chronically on my hands and feet. I would medicate daily with the cortisone creams, and while I found some relief at the contact spots, invariably new cracks and irritations would return. It was frustrating and annoying; I thought I had nipped this condition in the bud. I wasn't getting any answers from doctors and dermatologists. My visits were always met with the same results: a new prescription for steroid cream. I was back to my childhood days, where eczema was treated as an incurable, lifelong condition. I was really frustrated, mostly at the fact that I was shrugged off and not listened to. I felt unheard, as if I was just another cog in the wheel of the medical community.

I soon realized that I would have to take matters into my own hands if I wanted to try anything new or see any results. I started to consult with a naturopath, first looking at my diet and other ways to support my skin. I had many food allergies when I was younger, so I was used to seeing how my body reacted to foods. It was a long shot; I hadn't changed much in my diet over the past ten to twenty years and I ate fairly healthily. I couldn't rationalize why my skin would react now and why the eczema would return and not get better, even when how I lived hadn't changed. It was a start, though, and a place from which I was willing to jump off.

I did some blood work to isolate possible triggering foods and the results were extremely upsetting at first. Almost everything that I enjoyed in my diet seemed to now be off limits: from the obvious gluten and dairy to everyday fruits and vegetables. It was almost impossible for me to follow the restrictions diligently without major disruption to our family's meals, so I decided to focus on mostly gluten- and dairy-free, the two most common triggers for inflammation. Perhaps removing them would help reduce any strain on my body that could be encouraging the eczema.

That was August 2015. By January 2016, after months of not seeing much improvement, I knew that I needed to find another way to fix the problem. I turned to the Internet.

Chapter 7

DOWN THE RABBIT HOLE

I am a fiend for information. Give me a problem and I will attack it with gusto, researching as much as I can to help conceptualize the issue. This was a very useful characteristic when I was working at my corporate event planning job, where it was imperative for me to know every detail, every angle, and arm myself with all the information in order to speak with authority to executives, staff, and vendors. But this advantageous business trait wasn't necessarily the best attribute when searching for something personal. It would often send me down a rabbit hole of information-gathering, tangling me up in strings and links and causing me to lose many hours. When I first started googling about eczema, pages and pages of what it was, how an outbreak could occur, and various treatment options all popped up. The same repetitive information that I was told as a child was continually regurgitated in article after article, paper after paper. The more I looked, the less I found that was new or innovative or, quite frankly, helpful.

Until one search yielded a very different response. Whether as a result of all the hours I had researched or by some form of Divine intervention, in front of me was information on something called topical steroid addiction. Now this was interesting.

Topical steroid addiction (TSA) occurs with the systemic overuse of topical steroid creams, traditionally used to treat skin conditions like eczema. Patients who experience eczema symptoms, mostly small rashes or abrasions on the skin, are prescribed a mild form of corticosteroid cream. The cream is applied to the affected area and some relief is found. As new outbreaks occur, the efficacy of the cream wanes, and the skin doesn't respond to treatment. Invariably, a higher dose of steroid cream is prescribed in order to get the skin back under control. Once this is abused, again the skin doesn't respond. The cycle of upping the dosage continues.

By this time, the skin has become addicted to the application of steroid cream. Unaware of this, the patient continues to use cream to manage and soothe flares or outbreaks. However, there is some belief that now the steroid cream actually *induces* eczema rather than providing relief from it. The only way to break this cycle is to stop using all steroid creams cold turkey. This is an unconventional and some may think radical idea, but it's a concept that has some growing traction.

Dr. Marvin Rapaport, a dermatologist based out of Beverly Hills, is the pioneer behind this idea. His website explains steroid addiction, and subsequently topical steroid withdrawal (TSW), and what to expect when you cease using steroid cream[1]. I spent hours poring over this information, trying to get as solid a grasp as I could on what he was presenting. It was a lot to take in and something that seemed so far-fetched that I was having trouble wrapping my head around it all.

How could a cream, prescribed to me as a baby, and doled out with equal nonchalance at every doctor's appointment over my lifetime, be the cause of so much pain and discomfort? How could doctors and dermatologists, whom I trusted and went to for advice, have so willingly written scripts for something that could do so much damage, essentially trapping my body in a cycle that I would have no knowledge or understanding of and one in which couldn't be easily ended? Not once in my thirty-nine years had anyone raised a flag as to the possibility of addiction or long-term side effects: this just wasn't a conversation that anyone was having. The idea that what I was using to help my skin was actually the cause of all the damage was almost too difficult to accept. This Dr. Rapaport must be a little radical.

My natural curiosity didn't let me stop there, though. Something was nagging at me, tugging at me. As much as I didn't want to fall prey to this far-out idea, I couldn't let it go completely. Why would this reputable doctor, with nothing to gain, risk ridicule and disbelief in an apparent effort to help people? Radical ideas usually stem from some desire to control or harm others, but Dr. Rapaport's idea, at the core, seemed to be there to help those who were

1 Red Skin Syndrome, Dr. Marvin Rapaport, www.red-skin-syndrome.com

suffering. A life preserver in the drowning waters. Maybe this idea was not so radical after all.

For the next week or so, I changed my search from "cures for eczema" to "topical steroid withdrawal" and the results were staggering. Blog posts, articles, and images abounded, confirming that this really was a thing. Each new page I found, each new story I stumbled upon, broke my heart and soon I was left feeling deflated, heartbroken, and sad. So much suffering and so much pain. The lengths that some had endured in their skin battle because of topical steroid addiction and then withdrawal were harrowing. Some stories were too difficult to read, some images too disturbing to look at.

But there were also stories of success. Of triumph. Of freedom. Some were offered through Dr. Rapaport, some from other research. It was clear that if you had the grit, stamina, and determination to accept that the steroids were doing the harm and creating the eczema, you could persevere . If you had the courage to stop using the steroids and enter withdrawal, you would heal. For me now, the question was: Can I do this? Even more than that: Do I have the courage to do it?

Later that evening as Andre and I were settling in to watch our shows, I told him about everything I had found. He didn't seem discouraged; in fact, he just said, "You've got to do it."

Did I, though? I mean, did I really have to do it? Yes, my hands and feet were an annoyance, but did I want to propel myself down the path of uncertainty to try to heal them? Was what could potentially be months of the unknown be worth more than the acceptance of my skin not being perfect? While there was no definitive timeline for healing, the general rule was about one month of healing for every year that you used steroids, whether consistently or intermittently. If I decided to stop using steroids right then, it would be about forty months of withdrawal for me, close to three and a half years, with no real guarantee that I would be fully healed or even whether this path would be the right and true one for me. I had read the success stories, those who had come through on the other side, but I'd also read about the difficulties and setbacks. Was this really an undertaking that I needed, or even really wanted to endure?

I knew I had Andre's unwavering support, but I needed a little time to think about what this would mean for me and our family. Over the next few days I marinated the idea: while there were numerous reasons for not forging this path, for some reason it just felt right. I couldn't explain it. Even with all the images of the torment that others went through, even with the knowledge of how long, at a minimum, my healing would be, I couldn't shake the feeling that *it was just right*. I was destined to be in this moment, taking this new journey. I had this understanding, this knowing, that everything up to this point had prepared me for this health journey. It was time for me to take control of my life, to steer my body into health, and I felt a resolve and determination that I could do it.

Chapter 8

AND SO IT BEGINS

In January 2016, I stopped using all my prescription steroid creams. I should have recorded the actual date in my calendar, but I didn't, so I don't have any permanent notation of when my life took a completely new direction. At the time, I didn't realize how significant the day would be, but it was the first step in healing my body.

My eczema was only on my hands and feet at this point, and it had been that way consistently for about a year or so. While it had been worse at times, generally it was just an annoyance and a bit uncomfortable. During the previous year as I'd searched for a way to fully heal the eczema, I was still able to live normally. My decision to stop all steroid creams wasn't because of debilitating skin but rather as part of my quest to get healthy throughout my body and to help set me on a better path that didn't rely on creams or ointments to calm my eczema. In the first few weeks of the new year and into February, I actually saw a slight improvement. I was able to walk a bit better, and my hands weren't as cracked and sore as they had been the month previous. I remember meeting friends for dinner in late February or early March and gleefully telling them how miraculous the body is in knowing how to heal itself. While I had prepared myself for some difficult moments, I was almost smug in my initial discussions about my progress. I think I had an underlying thought that because I lived relatively healthily, and because I was never on heavy doses of cortisone, maybe I would just sail through with minimal issues.

The pictures and descriptions of the withdrawal symptoms I'd found during my research were both horrifying and terrifying, but somehow in my mind, naively, I didn't believe that my recovery would be that bad. It was true that I'd used steroids for a long time, including daily inhalers to control my asthma, but I'd never used injectable steroids or more harsh ones like prednisone and I'd never been hospitalized for my condition. I was hopeful, based on my initial response, that my withdrawal would be manageable and soon I would be able to live steroid-free.

By March 2016, I was in the beginning stages of what would become my life for the next four-plus years. Seemingly almost overnight, my body started to transform into something unrecognizable. My skin began to get progressively worse. I had severe redness on my arms and legs, something referred to in topical steroid withdrawal (TSW) circles as red sleeve syndrome (RSS), where the arms are beet red from the shoulder down, stopping at the wrists.

Red blotches also began to appear on my torso and my skin was very, very itchy.

I had thought, of course, that I was ready for this. I had researched and mentally come to terms with the fact that I was likely going to experience discomfort and worsening skin for some time before it got better. I thought I was prepared. I wasn't. No amount of research could have primed me for the depths to which the withdrawal process would take me. I was starting to see that I had underestimated the lengths I would need to go to in order to heal, and that I was unbelievably naive in my hopes for a quick or manageable recovery. By May, I was deep in the throes of massive withdrawal. The hell had begun.

For TSW and RSS patients, the healing journey is unpredictable. The intensity and length of TSW varies for each person. Some who have used steroid creams for a long time find the cycling through healing takes years. Others find relief and normalcy within a few months. There is no set timeline and while symptoms are universal, the intensity and magnitude of each varies widely among patients. I was in the fortunate position that I was at home. Other than attending to my daughter's needs, I didn't have to go anywhere or see anyone. I didn't have to worry about getting to a job on time or meeting a work deadline. This condition can wreak havoc on many people's lives, to the point where some can't work at all and have to rely on family for help. Many sufferers can't find support and have to take a leave of absence from their jobs, seeing their income dwindle and their associations shrink. Some are bedridden. All are desperate.

Desperate for answers, desperate for relief, but mostly desperate to live.

It's difficult to adequately describe the insidious nature of TSW. It comes on hard and strong at times and then whimpers softly for a while. It lures you into thinking you've won, only to shoot you back to ground zero in a heartbeat. It mocks you and teases you. But, most of all, it hurts you.

The physical pain is something I had never experienced before in my life, nor was it something I could have adequately prepared for. My skin became its own entity, one that I obsessed over. This obsession was different than from my earlier years suffering with eczema. While I thought constantly about my skin when I was younger, now, not only did I think about my skin non-stop, but I couldn't think of anything else. It was like my earlier youthful obsessions were magnified and now, my skin was totally consuming my thoughts in constant, repetitive and unhealthy ways. I couldn't escape its torture, for that really is what TSW is: it is torture.

On a physical level, my body would cycle through unimaginable stages. Initially, a body part would ooze: a yellowy, at times pungent, liquid that would stain sheets and make it difficult to wear clothes. The skin would be red, sometimes beet red, with immense heat emanating from it. Next, the ooze would eventually subside and enter the crusting stage. A tissue-paper layer of skin would develop that pulled so tightly, physical movement was difficult. Each step or turn would elicit a pulling and ripping so painful that I often wished for the burning, oozing stage to return. This would next lead into the skin shedding cycle where evidence of my skin would be everywhere; sheets, furniture, dark surfaces and floors. While not physically painful at this point, the itch would be unbearable and the constant visual reminder of skin flakes at every turn was demoralizing. My body would experience all these stages at different times in different areas, but the cycle would continue: ooze, crust, shed, repeat. In all, I think I likely shed and reproduced my skin more than a dozen times.

At the same time, my body was learning how to regulate itself after a lifetime of suppressing its natural composition. Topical steroids (also referred to as corticosteroids) are a synthetic drug produced to mimic the hormones that are naturally produced by the adrenal glands in the body.[2] When the body is faced with an allergic event, it naturally produces inflammation - causing chemicals and these are released into the body. They cause the blood vessels to widen and other inflammatory substances to arrive and this results in the affected area becoming itchy and swollen.[3] When applied topically, the steroid is absorbed into the skin and prevents these chemicals from being released into the body and acts as a powerful anti-inflammatory and immune suppressant. Over time, the body can become lazy, allowing the steroid cream to do the work of what the naturally producing chemicals would have done. Now, when the corticosteroid use is stopped, the body goes into hyper-drive, looking for this anti-inflammatory assistance while being thrust into an action it is unprepared

2   Topical Steroids 101, ITSAN, itsan.org

3   Topical corticosteroids ,netdoctor ,netdoctor.co.uk

for. My life-long use of topical steroids meant that when I stopped using them, my body's natural responses had been suppressed for so long, it didn't know what to do. I would have cold sweats while emanating so much heat that I couldn't find relief. I would experience so much fatigue that I couldn't really do anything in the day. I would also experience extreme nerve pain and a deep, deep itch that was so intense and painful it would cause me to mentally break down. I was quite literally living within my own physical and personal hell that I couldn't shake off and leave behind. I couldn't escape the pain and the humiliation; I had to carry it with me everywhere.

My body also changed shape and appearance. I became swollen, suffering eczema in my legs and ankles, and an increase in my waist size. I looked old. As the fluid worked its way through my body, I'd go from puffy to saggy, stretched to loose. My daily routine involved hours of slathering my skin with zinc oxide to help mitigate the ooze, wrapping my various body parts in gauze, and finding clothes that hid these extra layers as best I could. Mirrors became the enemy, as looking at myself didn't just make me sad, it made me scared. The visual reminder that I didn't have control over my appearance, no way to tighten the sagging skin, no way to brighten the ashy colour, no way to clear the angry red flares, was too much to bear. The hardwood floors and dark surfaces of my home constantly taunted me with powdery, flaky skin everywhere, and my bedsheets mocked me with yellow ooze-stained and blood-laden sheets. I felt like I was rotting.

As the days, months, and years passed, I continued to inhabit a body that I didn't recognize. While I was at times amazed at its ability to heal and repair itself in spots without intervention, I was also repulsed by how grotesquely it could morph into something that I didn't feel connected to or even a part of. My skin hung in ways that aged me more than ten years. Called "elephant skin," as fluid left a particular body part, the skin would sag and lay in rings, similar to the look of the skin of elephants.

It was actually quite easy to isolate myself from the rest of humanity and hide my condition from my friends. I found that my life was all consumed by my condition. When I went out, when I socialized, when I traveled were all dependent on how I was feeling and what level of pain my skin was at. I didn't have much of a life outside my home, it too feeling like both a refuge and a prison. It gave me comfort, privacy, and calm. But it also isolated and trapped me. I was a slave to a master whose intentions were not clear. My life was dictated by the whims and follies of a fickle condition seeming to mock me at every turn.

I was dealing with such great polarity at that time. There was so much physical and emotional pain, so much disruption and destruction of everything in my life, yet I had a feeling in my heart that I had made the right decision. Even though I was living an existence that provided no comfort or joy, I never questioned that I wasn't where I was supposed to be. I never considered starting with the creams again, to throw in the towel and just live with my condition forever. I couldn't go there. It is difficult to explain, but it was something deep within my core being that knew I had to go through this, that there was something at the end of this that I needed to get to. No matter how painful, embarrassing, humiliating, and debilitating the process was, I knew it was what I had to do.

But even knowing, in my heart, in my soul, that I was where I needed to be, it sometimes wasn't enough to help me through. I loathed myself and I couldn't understand why my husband stood by me in all my decrepitude. Since I could barely look at myself, I couldn't understand how he could bear to exist with a human who looked and acted nothing like the person he'd married. His fun loving, positive wife had been replaced by a depressed shell who would cry every night and not be able to be physically touched. Because touching did hurt, and at times I wasn't able to hug or hold Sydney either. I had never hated myself so much as I did in those days. I was turning into a person I didn't recognize, both physically and emotionally.

Because there was another side to this horrific process: the mental torture, which I didn't anticipate would be as severe as it turned out to be. On an intellectual level, I knew that going through any transformative or traumatic experience would involve some mental health challenges. I knew that there would be good days and bad, ups and downs. What I didn't anticipate, though, was the severity of those extremes and how out of my control they would be. I couldn't prepare for the emotional and mental depths that I would plunge into, or for the desperation I would feel.

The mental and emotional parts were just as difficult for me as the physical part. Every emotion I was feeling throughout the process was so counter to how I viewed life and how

I had lived my life that it left me off balance and distraught. When faced with adversity or disappointment in the past, I use to validate the feelings and then pick myself up. When I was emotional, I used to allow the emotion to happen, wallow in it a bit, and then see tomorrow as a new start and a new day. I had lived my life with a glass-half-full mentality so to feel so emotionally and mentally out of control was terrifying to me. Early on, the depression and despondency were so intense that I would be immobile on the couch in tears for hours. I lacked any type of motivation to do anything—even getting up to make lunch proved difficult. I was able to barely keep it together to ensure that Sydney had everything she needed for school and I would muster up the courage as best I could to make sure she got to school, appointments, and any activities, but it was a thin veil.

I cried every night with Andre. I cried most days by myself alone in the house. I developed a rage I couldn't explain. Huge angry outbursts would happen for no reason. Even though I knew I was overreacting and out of control, I was incapable of dialling it down or stopping. I caused so much pain in my little family of three that often Andre and Sydney didn't know which Allyson they would encounter each day. Coupled with the physical restrictions, I felt trapped by something out of my control. At times, I questioned whether I would ever be free of the torment, if I would ever be happy again. I had fleeting thoughts of whether life would be that bad if I weren't here anymore. For the first time in my life, I was really scared. Scared of who I was, scared of what my new life might look like, and scared that I was lost forever.

Chapter 9

FINDING SUPPORT

It is important to understand that not only do patients with TSW experience tremendous physical and psychological pain, but they have very little support available to help them cope. Most dermatologists view eczema as a chronic condition, one that is stimulated or aggravated by various triggers. According to the National Eczema Association, there are seven types of eczema with *atopic dermatitis* being the most common effecting close to ten million children and over sixteen million adults in the United States alone.[4] Exact numbers are not easily found for Canada, but it is assumed that about 17% of the Canadian population suffer from some form of eczema. Atopic dermatitis is caused by something within the body that has a tendency to become

---

4   Atopic Dermatitis, National Eczema Association, www.nationaleczema.org

inflamed, possibly because of imbalances in the body composition or because of other triggers like stress. *Contact dermatitis* is another common type of eczema caused by a trigger outside the body, such as various substances that irritate the skin, like soap, detergents, or makeup. As a child, I was diagnosed with atopic dermatitis, but I also experienced flares from contact dermatitis. I had all sorts of triggers, including but not limited to dairy, eggs, nuts, laundry detergents, all animals (but cats and horses being the most severe), cut grass, dust, mould, and various other environmental elements like trees, weeds, pollens. The list seemed endless. As an adult, I outgrew some of those allergies, but an outbreak could be triggered without a real correlation to anything.

In my experience, the easy answer for dermatologists was to prescribe topical steroid creams to treat an outbreak. As I mentioned in the previous chapter, topical steroids work to decrease inflammation that is a result of various skin conditions like psoriasis and eczema. Administered through creams and gels, the steroid is applied to the skin to reduce inflammation and constrict blood vessels just under the surface of the skin. The creams vary greatly in potency, and most are prescribed to be used for short periods of time. Combined with other alternative methods to soothe the skin, like wearing cotton clothing and taking oatmeal baths, it has been generally believed that using steroid creams topically is an effective way to treat the symptoms of eczema. While most medical organizations, including the Mayo Clinic, detail that steroid creams are not a cure for eczema but merely a mechanism to treat the symptoms, many dermatologists advocate the use of steroids without much education for the patient. Things may be different now, but as a child, neither I nor my mom were counselled on the side effects of using the creams long term, nor on the need to possibly look at healing the body from within in order to reduce inflammation and taper the use of creams over time.

In fact, even as late as the summer of 2015, my referral to a dermatologist to treat the chronic eczema on my hands and feet was met with exactly the same conclusion: use topical steroid cream to reduce the inflammation, and after a few days the symptoms would resolve themselves. Even as an adult, as I asked questions or probed further, I did not receive any advice or information on possible side effects or symptoms to be aware of while using the creams. It was as common as prescribing an antibiotic, a veritable revolving door, a quick-in, quick-out scenario.

That's what started to frustrate me the most. Growing up, I just did what the doctors told me to do and didn't question things too much. This wonder cream would help take my eczema away for a while, and surely the dermatologists wouldn't advocate something that wasn't safe. I blindly followed like a cult member, brainwashed into thinking there wasn't anything wrong with my treatment plan. But as an adult, I started to question more, and I started to notice the flippancy in which doctors and dermatologists regarded my condition. Whenever I made an appointment for prescription renewal, no one spent any time learning more about my circumstances. They didn't question how long I'd been using steroid creams, what other steroids I'd been using (in my case, a twice-daily inhaled steroid to treat asthma), or probed for information about my lifestyle. They didn't question my diet, my sleeping habits, my exercise routine, or my stress levels. A quick look at my skin and steroid creams were the only answer. And a swift one at that.

As I became more concerned about a healthier lifestyle, specifically because I wanted to start our daughter off on the right foot, I began to look more closely at my own health, trying to connect the scattered dots of my rocky, inexplicable health issues. Why wasn't any doctor or dermatologist concerned that a thirty-something-year-old woman was still having outbreaks of eczema? Why didn't anyone ask me questions? Why couldn't they think of a more natural approach to treating my skin irritations?

I found it increasingly difficult to get a sympathetic ear or an alternative viewpoint. At my appointments I started to feel more like a number and less like a human. I was just one of many who were experiencing a chronic, lifelong condition, and any special attention was more of an annoyance rather than an opportunity to try something different.

As I delved deeper into my research on eczema and ultimately topical steroid addiction, I came across more and more stories of people around the world who experienced the same thing. Interestingly, I found these accounts through various support and advocacy groups that had been formed primarily because people weren't getting answers from the medical community.

At the same time, I understood it. Faced with severe cutbacks, lack of funding, an increased demand on the health system, even the admired Canadian healthcare system was overwhelmed. I didn't fault my doctors or dermatologists for not thinking outside the box. The time pressures and exhausted resources meant that the doctors I saw were only doing what they believed was the only solution. I was increasingly frustrated, yes. But more so with a broken healthcare system that left many, including doctors, unsupported.

I realized that I would have to weather this storm alone. While I hitched myself to naturopathic doctors and alternative treatments here and there, generally I had to find the resolve within myself to keep going and stay the course. When a flare crippled me from participating meaningfully in my life, I had to remind myself that this was the course, this was the path to healing and that something had pushed me to make this decision. I needed to believe in myself more than I had ever been challenged to do so before.

Chapter 10

IT'S HARD TO BELIEVE

When I took moments to take stock of everything, I still grappled with disbelief. Even after all my research and seeing other survivors and reading their stories, I had to admit that I didn't fully believe that I would ever be that bad. Using steroid creams had been such an integral part of my life that there was still a part of me that couldn't connect how something that was prescribed to me as an infant could ever produce such a ferocious response in my body. I had prepared for the discomfort and went into it with my eyes open and was honest with myself on what I may encounter. But, deep down, there was that niggling feeling that it just wasn't true. I had been shown the evidence before, but like many of the doctors and friends and family, it was as if my brain couldn't process the truth.

Throughout my entire journey, I had doubt. Doubt about whether this was the best course of action. Doubt about whether I would actually experience the kind of turmoil that many others had. Doubt that what I was trying to do to support my body was making everything worse. I too found myself questioning whether food caused a flare, whether having that glass of wine was prohibiting the healing, whether exercising too much triggered an outbreak, or whether not exercising enough didn't promote positive endorphins.

So much doubt.

Even after four years and being able to see the healing with my own eyes, I still had doubt when a new flare would materialize. Had I done something to encourage this new flare? Were my thoughts racing again? Was withdrawal even real, and was what I had been doing and enduring really making any difference at all? How could I see improvement and then be flung back into the thick of things? Was there ever really going to be an end to all this?

That was the real insidious part of this condition. It had no pattern, no real trajectory that I could trace. After four years, I was still dealing with the setbacks and the dryness and the ooze. The pendulum would swing one way and I would see relief, only to swing again and bring on another flare. Certain areas of my body would take forever to heal, while others would heal quickly and permanently. It was exhausting and infuriating and so disheartening.

But I had become a believer, and it angered me. The thing I have to make perfectly clear is that topical steroid addiction is real and topical steroid withdrawal is very much a true affliction. Every single person I listened to in my support group, every single story I read: we were all the same. The same symptoms, the same pain, the same uncertainty, albeit all in varying degrees, but the same story nonetheless. It was so important to me to somehow tell this story so that others would believe it too. I understood how crazy it all seemed to those who weren't sufferers. I got how unbelievable all this looked and sounded. Because it *was* crazy and unbelievable. To think that something that is told will help support us actually destroys us is unconscionable. To think that babies and children are given a substance that promotes unknown addiction is almost inhumane.

But it *is* real. It's happening all the time and with more frequency. Even mild amounts of steroid creams are available without a prescription at pharmacies. Products made by Gold Bond, Exederm and Polysporin, for example, contain 1% Hydrocortisone and are available and marketed as safe alternatives for eczema relief. By using terms like, eczema relief, hypoallergenic, and promoting fast relief from itching, inflammation and rash, the general public is unknowingly administering products they believe are safe, often without concern for duration of use. Many beauty products also contain some form of steroid and there are so many that are unknowingly using products that could cause so much pain in the future. We must be diligent in understanding what is in our health products and what we are allowing into our bodies.

But most importantly, we have to recognize that addiction to steroid creams can happen to anyone and the consequences are devastating. Even mild and short-term use can cause an addiction, and we must be able to separate what is actually a skin condition from a reaction to the withdrawal symptoms of ceasing the use of steroid creams. So many people I read about would experience severe skin reactions while using steroids that many doctors and even the patients themselves believed that it was actually a worsening of the condition and not attributed to the "cure." As the efficacy of the cream lessened, more potent creams were prescribed.

The takeaway in this scenario, though, is that the more potent medications only exacerbate the situation, causing an increase in the dependency of and a greater reliance on the creams. It becomes a cycle of the body building a tolerance to a cream, so finding relief at that potency becomes impossible, so a higher dosage is given that then creates a greater dependency on that cream, which invariably over time stops working and higher dosages are prescribed, and so on. The steroid creams do not address the root problem and, in fact, create whole new problems of topical steroid addiction and steroid-induced eczema, where the treatment is actually worsening the condition. That's what happened to me, without a doubt. My decades use of steroid creams as well as an inhaled steroid for asthma created a perfect storm inside my body, where a battlefield was always raging. It was a war I couldn't see. It was my body fighting for autonomous control over its own system, only to be losing that battle to a foreign entity introduced from the outside. And that entity now had control. It had control over every aspect of my body: from temperature moderation to its ability to produce its own cortisol.

The skin is the body's largest organ, and what we put on our skin is absorbed and transmitted through every cell in our body. Our blood vessels are wonderful little worker bees, but in the case of topical steroids, they deliver those toxins wonderfully around the entire body, even if it's only needed in one spot. This is what we need to be aware of.

We have to stop the use of topical steroids for the treatment of skin conditions and look to alternative ways to heal. Whether it's time, diet, exercise, sleep, meditation, or a combination of all of those and more, the need to remove topical steroids as a treatment is not only imperative, it's crucial.

I'm not a doctor, chemist, or pharmacist. I don't have any medical training or full knowledge of how anatomy works. But I've learned to understand it a bit more and I've learned to become an advocate for my own health. We all have a right to have dominion and domain over our own bodies, but that is only accomplished if we educate ourselves and take notice of what works and what doesn't. I am only speaking about my individual experience and one that I know to be true. The body does not need topical steroids to treat any skin condition. The body does not require the use of topical steroids to soothe, calm, or heal skin conditions, especially eczema. There is a time and a place for medicine and there are many cases where a steroid works and is warranted, but not in creams and ointments to treat eczema.

And definitely not in easily accessible over-the-counter products at pharmacies and drugstores. Definitely not in makeup products or skin products. Read labels, scour ingredients, and be an advocate for your own health. No one else needs to experience the unique and excruciating degree of suffering caused by topical steroid withdrawal.

Chapter 11

A DIFFERENT APPROACH

In the summer of 2016, I decided that I needed to take a more natural approach to my health and think more seriously about how I was treating my body. I had dabbled in more restrictive eating early on in my journey and I was ready to explore that again to find, at the very least, an alternative strategy to the medical help that I had relied on in the past. Initially, much of what I tried were home remedies that I could do myself. I prepared a cream of shea butter with essential oils that included, rosemary, frankincense, lavender, geranium, and wintergreen. It was the only thing that I could apply to my skin that didn't cause any burning or major irritation. In the early months I spent hours researching various herbal tinctures and essential oils that could help heal or provide a remedy to calm my skin. I tried various combinations of oils, different carrier agents, varying strengths and potencies. It was an exercise in experimentation but I was eager to find anything that would work. All of the queries I would look at in the support group I followed on Facebook would provide numerous suggestions on what could work and what others had tried in order to ease the burning and itching of the skin. There were always hundreds of ideas as no one treatment seemed to work for everyone. It was clear that everyone reacted differently to treatments and there was definitely no one size fits all solution. Most tried something for awhile until it started to irritate and then they would try something else. For me, eventually everything I tried irritated, burned and itched my skin and I had to stop using anything at all.

I really only found true relief in my daily Epsom salt baths. I was unable to take showers for about two to three years while going through the withdrawal. The shower pressure would irritate my skin and it just seemed to exacerbate the situation. I would be in more pain after a shower then sometimes I was before. The Epsom salt baths were my only means of cleaning and they also provided some relief to all the pain. My nightly ritual would revolve around peeling the bandages and gauze pads from various parks of my body, fill the tub with copious amounts of epsom salts and soak for over an hour. In the really horrible months, I would often take two to three of these baths a day in order to find some relief. Sometimes they would sting and burn at first, especially if there were open wounds, but eventually the skin would soften and I could peel the skin from my body without damaging the skin beneath that was trying to heal. I relished these nights.

Much more than a relaxing experience, they were the only thing that helped me keep my sanity in check at times. For at least one hour a day, I could escape the incessant, continuous burning and aching of my body. And I felt a strange sense of control and dominance when I would peel the skin from my body and watch it swirl in the bath water. Like I was at that moment the one taking over, the one that had domain over my body and not the other way around. I felt a tremendous release after I completed my baths, like a cathartic healing of my mind and body.

In addition to my healing home remedies, I realized that I should maybe seek out some professional advice and treatment. I was skeptical and very adverse at this point with medical doctors so I decided to reach out to a naturopathic doctor I had seen interviewed on a blog I followed. He had experienced some topical steroid withdrawal symptoms as a child so I thought he may have a deeper understanding of the condition and what I was going through than what my family doctor was able to understand. He was in high demand, with a waiting list no shorter than three months. Luckily for me, my at-home life without work commitments meant that I could be available should a cancellation arise. I was put on a waitlist and within a week, I was able to get in to see him.

I saw him regularly at first as we worked through rebalancing me from the inside. I was prescribed a specific protocol for natural supplements, which included a vitamin B complex, digestive enzymes, probiotics and fish oils to name a few. I was also challenged to change some of my thought patterns. Concepts like; learn to say no (setting boundaries doesn't make me a bad person), know that good enough is good enough (there is no perfect, only practice) and know that I am a guide not a God (don't take on other people's problems as my own), were daily reminders I could say to myself to reset and restart my thoughts. I maintained a dairy-free, gluten-free diet and avoided pseudo-grains like quinoa as well as rice, corn and oats. These additional foods contain compositions that can mimic gluten so we decided to avoid them in the initial stages of my treatment. Within about six months, I did see progress on my hands and feet with less cracking and more improvement in the texture and appearance of the skin. Whether the improvement was directly attributable to my visits with my naturopathic doctor or simply due to time is difficult to say, but I do believe that supporting the body from within helped to provide a better foundation for healing.

Over the course of about three years, I would schedule follow-up appointments for every three months or so. During that time, I would have wonderful moments of reprieve, where my body would be in remission. I would also have extremely challenging times as the toxins released themselves from every part of my body and I would enter into the ooze, crust, flake cycle again. After about three years, I could tell that my naturopath was getting frustrated as to why I was still having problems with my skin. I didn't blame him, though; it *was* difficult to comprehend. For doctors, whether naturopathic or medical, it is in their nature, training, and experience to anticipate that their patients will see changes or results from the remedies for their health issues. The fact that I kept cycling through flares and healing was baffling and difficult for many to wrap their heads around, my doctors included. It got to the point that when I asked why I still wasn't healed, he would shrug his shoulders and say he really didn't know.

Much of my work with the naturopath centred around what my body wasn't producing enough of or what it was producing too much of. Whether it be certain digestive enzymes I needed to add, or a treatment to counter too much yeast in my system, we focused primarily on resetting the balance in my body. As I mentioned, food was also a key component in my treatment plan. Avoidance of certain triggers was key, and flares and outbreaks were often attributed to inflammatory foods or behaviours, like consuming too many night-shade vegetables, gluten, pseudo grains, sugar or alcohol or not allowing the body to get enough sleep. To some degree, I agree with much of that and at least initially, the more I could help reduce inflammation, the better my healing would be.

When I followed all the aspects of my treatment plan and was *still* experiencing difficult flares, I know it became confusing for my doctor to understand. There is always a cause-and-effect, so if my body wasn't healing with treatment, there must've been another cause that was hindering improvement. What is so difficult to relay to doctors and specialists about topical steroid withdrawal is that there is no way to attribute the healing cycle to anything in particular. There is no definite trigger, there is no guaranteed solution. I was learning that nutritional support was imperative but the body was going to heal when it decided it was ready to heal. The toxins were going to take their time, and the body didn't have a stopwatch for when it would begin to function normally again. The cause-and-effect scenario just doesn't exist with TSW.

When my naturopath felt that it had to be cause-and-effect—too much wine, splurging on gluten, for example—I would agonize over what I ate and drank. If I flared, I would go over my meals from the week prior to try to determine if I had done something wrong, or fell off the wagon somehow. Every time I relaxed with a glass of wine, I would stew about whether I was setting myself back in my healing journey. I would question what I was doing and admonish myself for not staying stricter to my regime. But I knew in my heart that any new flare was not related to food. After months and years of depriving myself and being cautious with what I ate, I was still faced with the unpredictability of what would happen with my skin. I did believe that the cleaner the diet I observed, the less inflammation I would have; and thus my body would have an easier time healing itself and getting rid of all the toxins. The less additional strain I put on my liver the better, so there was definite merit in supporting the whole body, inside and out. I was happy that I started to view my health and recovery from a different perspective, but ultimately I still held the systematic belief that where there is a problem, there has to be a cause. That just wasn't the case with me. So, while I continued with the practices and protocol that I followed and learned with my naturopath, I eased off on my appointments and decided to follow my natural instincts a bit more. I could hear my body whispering to me, and I knew I had to have more faith in what I was hearing.

Chapter 12

I'M FEELING A CHANGE

There will always be a "me before" and a "me after." While essences of myself remained consistent, I knew that after this experience I would never go back to who I used to be.

As I mentioned, very early in my journey I battled an aspect of this condition that I hadn't anticipated. Just as difficult but much more precarious than the physical healing was my mental wellbeing. I hadn't given credence to how quickly and unpredictably I could teeter off the edge and nosedive into depths I had never experienced before.

What was so frustrating about going through withdrawal was that I couldn't predict anything. I would ride the wave when my skin healed but would always be waiting on tenterhooks for the next storm to come. It was constantly on my mind, and my family and I were always on edge, not knowing when the next outbreak would occur and how severe it would be.

Because I have always been a glass half-full type of person, I have in the past been able to weather any emotional ups and downs. Don't get me wrong: I was, and still am, a deeply emotional person. I felt things to my core and would agonize for days, even months, about what someone thought of me or if I had said or done the right thing. I had a tendency to overthink and second-guess conversations, constantly worrying about offending people. I was so afraid of people not liking me. But as far as mental health, depression, despondency, hopelessness—those weren't things I ever had to deal with.

On some level, I had empathy for people who suffered because of their mental health. I am embarrassed to say that I didn't give it enough concern, though. While I could understand how someone's mental health could be compromised or how a particular life situation could encourage mental instability, I was callous in my internal reactions to such situations. I judged, thinking that all a person needed to do was to take control, seek counselling, and work on improving their mental health.

For those of us who go through TSW, our bodies have had to relearn how to do everything. Because the steroids suppress the body's natural abilities, when the drug is removed, the body kicks into hyper drive. Every nerve, organ, and body part goes through withdrawal; beyond the skin issues, my body had to learn how to do so many natural things. Regulating body temperature was a big one. Even in the summer months with humidity and heat, my body would be unable to control the cold sweats and constant shivering. My nerves needed to calm themselves and I would experience zingers, or quick jabs of nerve pain, as my body learned how to reconnect to itself. I would experience a deep itch, one that was never satisfied and gnawed at me constantly. And I had emotional and mental trauma.

The initial days were the hardest for me mentally. For the first six months or so, I would be plagued with a dark gloom. I was despondent and listless, roaming around my house in a perpetual fog, interspersed with crying jags. This state was foreign to me, somewhere that I was incapable of clawing myself out from. I knew I had to do something, I knew I had to help myself, but the weight of that held me back. Held me down.

I had always been a go-getter. Someone who was always up, doing things, trying new things, filling my day. Now I would find myself sitting on the couch, crying and getting deeper into a darkness that scared me. The only thing that kept me going was knowing that everything I was experiencing was temporary. I didn't know how temporary and for how long, but I intuitively knew that this wasn't my intended outcome. I would come through.

The "me before" always acknowledged that mental health was important, but the "me after" understood the real struggle and battle that is an all-day, every-day occurrence for many people. The "me before" had empathy but would silently judge; the "me after" had compassion and would openly embrace.

I wish it wasn't that way, though. I wish I didn't have to go through something in order to give it its full credence and weight. I wish I had had more compassion before, talked more, engaged more. I wish I had been able to understand

and evaluate without judgment or labels. But it was where I was then, and thankfully I have a much deeper understanding of mental health struggles and what many have to endure each day. I also have a deeper connection to figuring out how to embrace that which hinders you and finding ways to push through, become stronger, and persevere.

Early on, in the beginning, when I was finding it increasingly difficult to stay on level ground, I had to find a way to cope that didn't rely on dumping everything onto Andre each night. I had to find something to help me clear my head, centre my thoughts, and steer my emotions into a manageable direction.

As I mentioned, I was someone who liked to always be on the move. Much of that came from an angst that I couldn't understand. I literally could not sit around the house doing nothing. If I had time, I would be doing something. I liked to run errands on the weekend, checking things off my list as I went. Early on in my relationship with Andre, when we were first dating, this perpetual motion would cause some issues between us. Andre loved to relax and take it easy on the weekends, sleeping in, watching TV, puttering around. He would get increasingly annoyed at my impatience and I would get increasingly frustrated with his lack of oomph. We've had to work on that discord, but my health crisis has actually helped with that. So it was really difficult to be stuck in my home, doing virtually nothing, while the world whirred around outside. Not only was I dealing with feelings and emotions that were so intense, but I also had a serious case of guilt and unease at not being productive throughout my day. My mind was battling itself in all directions and that alone was not healthy. I needed to calm myself and do what Andre did and just relax.

My first go-to was the bookstore. I love, love, love books. I will read them back to back, often starting a new book right after I've finished reading the acknowledgements of the last one. As I was browsing through all types of self-help titles and metaphysical offerings, something about all these wonderful books spoke to me. Growing up Catholic, my family was religious when I was a child. We attended mass every Sunday, and my mom was a reader during mass. And while I technically believed in God and Jesus and saints, I didn't always connect with the religious aspect. I liked the rituals of mass and the community but not always with the interpretations or strict confines of the Catholic faith. I always felt much more spiritual. I felt connected to God, to a source in my soul. I didn't subscribe to the teachings often forced on you in the religious context, so perhaps this particular section of the bookstore was my soul connecting back to what I always felt.

I bought up a storm, grabbing books by Dr. Wayne Dyer, Louis Hay, and Mary Williamson alongside books about mindfulness, meditation, and natural remedies. It was all out of general interest, really. I wasn't sure if what I would find within the pages would be of any use, but I felt so drawn and connected to this selection that I had to just read them.

So I read and was enthralled, particularly with the subjects of meditation and mindfulness, the former being something that terrified my bubbling mind. Reading was my early therapy. It helped to calm my mind, and each new topic or concept intrigued me and gave me hope that I could push through.

As my mental state stood precariously on the edge, it was becoming clear to me that I had to take charge of the situation and find some way to shift the focus. At times I was sinking lower and lower into a feeling of hopelessness, and I felt in my soul that I had to do something before I was lost in that spiral forever.

I also found it unnerving that I felt so much anger, and even rage at times. I had never been an angry person—emotional, yes—but feelings of intense anger were not something I had experienced before. Now, during my withdrawal, the most insignificant things could set me off on a tirade. While I knew I was overreacting, I felt incapable of controlling myself. Some of my anger could absolutely be attributed to my failing health, the isolation I felt, and the disbelief that this was the situation I was in. But there was a tension sitting just below the surface that could erupt at any moment. It worried and scared me that I wasn't able to control the outbursts but also couldn't contain the ongoing wrath.

My body and my mind were trying to tell me something, and it was time that I paid attention and started to work on rebalancing myself as a whole being. If I didn't try to get a handle on my emotional and mental state now, I was afraid that it would overtake me and I wouldn't be the same person anymore.

Just as with my journey to heal my skin, this was a path I would likely have to traverse alone—but it was a necessity for me to do. For both my family and myself.

Chapter 13

ALTERNATIVE THERAPIES

At first, I didn't know where to start. In the past whenever things got stressful or I needed to calm myself down, I would go for a brisk walk outside. In my new reality, though, this wasn't possible. Some days I couldn't walk at all and I would find myself crawling through the house to get from the bed to the bathroom, down the stairs to the couch. It was difficult to move, so the physical release I used to get by walking needed to be replaced with something I could manage to do sitting or lying down.

Much of the reading and the books I had purchased revolved around the concept of quieting the mind and finding calm and peace through meditation. I was always hesitant about meditation—not because I didn't believe it worked, but more that I didn't think it would work for me. I liked to talk, especially to myself, and I often worked though difficult scenarios or hard times by talking myself through it and finding solutions. My mind was always racing, and the idea that I would need to sit and force my thoughts to cease was challenging for me. As I read more books and learned more about the practice, it was slowly becoming something that I felt I should try.

I started by trying to meditate for about 10 minutes a day. Initially, I would set myself up on the couch, open my guided meditation app, and try to focus on my breathing. The app's calming voice really helped me to start the process, and after a few weeks of trouble trying to get into the groove, I found that the quiet moments weren't as difficult to find. As with anything, practice was all that was needed to set my intention and help my mind stay focused. My reluctance and trepidation to start meditation were manifestations of my own mind: stumbling blocks I had put in my own way to prevent my initiation into this practice sooner. I had been talking myself out of it rather than gently encouraging myself to start. For the first three to four months of my withdrawal, I needed emotional support the most and I found that meditating helped to calm my nerves and refocus my thoughts. It didn't make the pain go away, or the itch stop, or the sadness dissipate—those were all things I needed to work through over time. What the mediation did do was almost arm me, providing me with the strength to persevere, to muster through, to hope. It guided me to a place where I started to see my existence as something much larger than just a physical one. Through quieting my mind and training my thoughts, I started to be filled with the feeling of something more. I didn't know what it was at the time, it was just a feeling, something niggling at me, but I knew that this thing I was going through, this torment I had accepted into my life, was there for a reason. I had made the decision for a reason. And it was going to be something big.

I continued my meditation, adding more time as my ability to remain still improved. When I was able to walk, I would take my practice outside and do walking meditations. Being outdoors had always soothed and calmed me. Walking had always been my joy. Because of the many months that my feet and skin were too severe to allow me to be outdoors, when the time came, I knew I needed to absorb and revel in the ability to do so.

Previously, walking had been an exercise in working out a problem, or venting my frustrations, but now it seemed to hold more sanctity. After months of hibernation, the world outside had so much more richness. I don't know if it was because something I had taken for granted before had been withheld from me for so long, or if I was actually changing my perspective, but nature bloomed more intensely. The colours were more vibrant, the sounds more joyous. I would spend my time walking, letting the deep blue of the sky and the marshmallow clouds feed my soul in a way that I had never experienced. It was joy.

My meditation practice helped me see from a different perspective. Much of what I had worried about before—all the anxieties that surrounded my health and the fear that I would never improve—were quieted when I meditated. For the moments that I allowed myself to go deeper within, I was able to keep those frightening thoughts at bay and shift to thoughts that focused on healing and positive outcomes.

I continued with the guided meditation because I found it the best way to help me centre my thoughts and progress without getting too sidetracked or out of the zone. It was still a process, though, and I struggled to get a good grasp on making each session as positive as I could.

When I first started meditating, so many thoughts would fly through my head. Many of my early attempts would first engage thoughts about all the things I needed to get done that day mixed with memories I really wished I could forget. Old relationships, old scenarios would come to light and I couldn't understand why my brain wouldn't let them go, almost *couldn't* let them go. My meditations would often find my regret getting stirred up, and it took a few months for me to be able to allow those thoughts, and all thoughts, to gently flow in and out without giving them any credence or importance. Through practice I was able to recognize that part of my process was to actually process; I would need to let go to move forward. I'll get into more on that later.

I also began to realize that I should find someone to talk to. I had been relying so heavily on Andre. While he was amazing and listened whenever I needed to talk and was patient when I needed to cry, it really wasn't healthy for either of us for him to be the only one I vented to. I needed to find a therapist.

I have always been a good listener, helping people with their problems or offering alternative perspectives. I really have a keen interest in learning about people and I guess my ability to put myself in someone else's position has been a strength that has allowed me to give counsel and an ear to whoever needed it. But it was never easy for me to share my own feelings. I was guarded about everything and I rarely sought the advice of anyone other than my parents or Andre. I never felt comfortable sharing. It's funny, I was always so eager for others to share with me, to help understand them more or to be a support, yet I never allowed the same in return. I was beginning to realize, though, that in order to heal and grow through this journey, I was going to have to open up.

My good friend Maha referred me to a therapist named Heather as she thought we would be a good fit. Heather was a holistic nutritionist, a therapist, and an empath, all fields that were fitting in with my growing interest in spirituality and Universal force.

When Heather and I first met, I was instantly drawn to her natural aura of warmth and connectedness. She had a brightness about her, and I felt totally safe and protected in her care. My reason for being there was, of course, driven by my skin. I wanted to find ways of pushing through the negative thoughts I had about my current situation and also dig a bit deeper to help calm my mind and stop my limiting beliefs.

Our first few sessions were intense and fascinating, uplifting and a bit scary. She set me on a path that I had really never intended: one that needed to be walked, but one that terrified me nonetheless. After our first session, it was clear that while I had compartmentalized my TSW into fixing my skin, I needed healing throughout my whole being. And if I only focused on my skin clearing and finding support through the physical journey, I wouldn't find peace, or comfort, or ever be living my best life. In such a short time opening myself up to my spiritual realm, I understood that who I was in the physical form was only one aspect of me. Until I connected with who I was at my core, my physical would always suffer in some way.

My body had been telling me this for years now really. From the first time I lost my voice, to the migraines, menstrual troubles and abscess, to finally my chronic skin condition, my spirit and soul were using my body to shake me up, to wake me up, and to push me to stand up and take charge of my life.

I quickly came to realize that what had started as a physical journey would ultimately become a spiritual one. I was sensing somehow that this wasn't just going to be about bringing my body back to full health—it was going to challenge me to look at and improve much more of myself, to cultivate my spiritual side as well. It was something that I hadn't anticipated, but as I worked through my meditation and leaned into my therapy more, I sensed that the real roadblock to my ultimate health could quite possibly be me.

Chapter 14

IT CONTINUES TO FLUCTUATE

It is easy for me to write all this now, after the fact, but when I was in the thick of things, I didn't have a full grasp on how much my mind and my body were connected. I plugged through, continuing with my meditation, therapy with Heather, and learning as much as I could about alternative ways to heal. Mentally, it was challenging at times. This stuff isn't easy. With each new day I was faced with more evidence that while time would eventually help to heal my body from the topical steroid addiction and withdrawal, if I wanted to continue to stay healthy, my mind would play a huge part. Theoretically, I got it; but in practice, I admit, I didn't always get it right.

Things kept progressing, though, and I did see an improvement in my skin overall during the winter of 2016. I started to really see some healing in my hands and feet and my mobility improved quite a bit as the beginning of

2017 approached. During the course of much of 2017 and into the first part of 2018, my body would go through one flare after another, some more intense than others. I was optimistic when a new flare would begin as I reminded myself that true healing really does happen if I just stay the course. My hands and feet were a great indication of what is possible when you persevere; what had been a physically debilitating and horrible time, was now in the past and I could walk again and get outside. My mood would shift dramatically as each flare prolonged and my resolve would sometimes waver, wondering if it could or would heal as well as my feet did. My arms and legs would go through the cycle, as would areas throughout my torso. Some flares would be over quickly, lasting a month or so in the ooze, dry, shed cycle, others for more than three months or so. It was a trying few years with so much physical and emotional upheaval but I did see improvements with the passage of time. Luckily, I did not have any outbreaks on my face, so I was still able to wear makeup and do my hair to make myself feel good. By January and February 2018, I thought I was through the worst of it.

Around the time of my birthday in June, the ooze started again—this time around my waist, thighs, and bum. It was upsetting because I had been free of the oozing for a good six months and I didn't want to go back there. However, I was confident, having experienced this before on other parts of my body, that it would subside and I would get through. It would just be a new cycle of ooze, dryness, repair.

At the beginning of June my mom called to take me out for a birthday lunch. Although I accepted, I didn't tell her that I was a little reluctant with my ooze. It was unpredictable whether it would be persistent or calm for the day, and I was finding it difficult to not let my anxiety and nerves get out of control. But I decided to just go for it and began the ritual that I hadn't had to do for some time; I lathered myself up with zinc cream, which helped to stop the ooze a bit, wrapped copious amounts of gauze and non-stick pads around the various areas, and put on a thicker pair of pants. We had a nice lunch, and I was able to forget a bit about my current state. When I returned home, though, it was clear to me that I really was entering another flare, possibly the most difficult one yet.

As June transitioned into July, I realized that the summer of 2018 would be my summer of forced leisure. Due to the parts of my body that were experiencing outbreaks, it was difficult to wear clothes. Underwear and waistbands would get stuck in my ooze and crusting and taking clothes off would rip my skin away. I spent most of the time in a housecoat, moping around the house. Sydney was away at camp for almost three weeks during that time, so the only thing I needed to do was make sure I got up and had something to eat.

When Andre returned home from work, we would order takeout or pick something up as I found it hard to get motivated to cook anything for dinner. I fell into somewhat of a depression again, at a loss as to how to stay positive. I spent the sun filled days in my living room, longing to be outside and finding what I could binge-watch on Netflix. I was so envious of everyone I could see out my windows; so carefree, so full of life, so energetic. My mind would find itself sinking back to those hopeless feelings again, the "what ifs" scenarios and general malaise. I was determined though, and even though it was mentally challenging again, I just continued to persevere and was buoyed as I started to see improvements in my skin. All the time spent laying low in the house and attempting to reduce any stress was helping and by the end of July, I had a reprieve of some of my symptoms. I still had some red skin patches and scabs where the skin was still trying to fully heal, but the ooze had stopped and the itching, burning skin was no longer plaguing me. We picked Sydney up at camp and we had so much fun being outdoors. I relished it.

And this reprieve couldn't have been better timing. In August, Andre, Sydney, and I were going on a trip with my parents to celebrate their fiftieth-wedding anniversary. Our trip to Budapest and Vienna had been in the works for more than a year and it was something that all of us were looking forward to. Andre and I are incredibly close with my parents and Sydney has a bond with her nana and grandpa that I am very grateful for. My dad was helping us with the cost of the trip and picking up the tab for our hotel, which was such a wonderful gesture and a testament to my parents' generous nature. To say that this trip was highly anticipated was an understatement.

The first few weeks of August saw a creeping of the symptoms back again. Small areas of my body began to ooze again, but it was manageable and the positive feelings I got from my earlier reprieve helped me to remember not to freak out and just go for the ride. The day before our flight, the ooze started again, more severe than it had been before. From my belly button to my upper thighs, it was like my skin was perpetually leaking. The smell of the ooze was pungent and gross, I felt sticky and hot. It was like a thin layer of my skin had been removed, exposing all the soft, vulnerable skin beneath, unshielded and unprotected. I was at a loss. The shear size of the area was overwhelming; in previous flares, it would be my legs, or my arms, or my torso. One area at a time, and I could compensate for the discomfort because I could tackle it one area at a time. Now it was one solid block of my body, right in the middle and everyday tasks, like sitting, walking and using the washroom became pain centres that sent shockwaves throughout my body. I covered my skin in non-stick padding and did the best I could to mitigate the oozing and cracking as much as possible. By the time we were supposed to leave for the airport, I was in complete hysterics. Why was this continuing to happen? By this point, I had been in TSW for over two and a half years, and I thought it would have been safe to plan a once in a lifetime trip with my family. I lost total control and was unable to keep my crying from escalating into a full blown attack. My crying upset Sydney and she started to cry too; soon a level of hysteria started to permeate. I couldn't bear to sit on a plane for more than eight hours: the mere thought of it sent me into panic mode. But cancelling meant I would ruin this event for all of us because Andre and Sydney refused to go without me. It was another reminder of how much TSW takes away from everyone, how much you have to sacrifice, and how much your family has to sacrifice. I took a moment to try to calm down, and I realized that I had to push through. My dad was experiencing some health issues himself. Not knowing if we would be able to take this type of trip again, I wanted to make sure we could have these memories, even if tinged by this flareup.

This flare was following the same pattern as the other flares on my body, but its location made it more difficult. Outbreaks around my waist, legs, and bum meant that walking was difficult and wearing clothes a tricky situation. I opted for casual, comfortable pants and top in cotton without a tight waistband, zippers or buttons. I wrapped the parts of my body I could reach in gauze, hoping to mitigate the ooze as best I could. By the time the three of us had made it from our house to the airport, through checkin and security, my clothes were completely soaked through. I don't think I had ever experienced a level of embarrassment and pure defeat as I did in that moment. When you body betrays you so thoroughly, when you are completely out of control of the situation, let me tell you, you become hopeless. Even with the prospect of a wonderful trip ahead, time with my family and the knowledge from my previous experience to help me, standing in an airport full of strangers, the acrid smell of ooze surrounding me, clothes drenched and sticky from all the fluid, I wanted nothing more than to close my eyes to the world, curl up and become invisible. But I had no choice and maybe that was the best thing really. I had to keep going I was here, we were on our way and I had to push through.

I found a sportswear store in the terminal and bought the first pair of leggings and long top I could find. I didn't try anything on, grabbing the largest pair I could find. In the washroom, I gently pulled the clothing from my skin, screaming silently in my head as I tried to extricate the fabric from the stickiness of ooze and crusting, put on my fresh clothes and stored my soiled pants in my carry on luggage. The plane ride to London was pure hell. I was unable to move most of my body, so moving positions at all caused a seizure of pain. I tried to sleep, distract myself with movies and chatting with Sydney and prayed constantly. When we landed and it was time to disembark to make our connecting flight, I noticed my seat was wet from all the ooze that had penetrated the gauze and my clothing. The embarrassment and humiliation was almost too much for me to bear and I tried to conceal my tears that threatened to escape my fragile self.

Our connecting flight was short and soon we were in Budapest and on our way to the hotel. It was so hot, a record heatwave in Europe that year and walking into the air conditioning of the hotel felt like luxury. I was depleted but grateful to finally be on solid ground and able to rest in comfort and peace. In our room, I wrapped myself in a housecoat and rested in bed while Andre and Sydney explored some of the city close by the hotel. I had sent them on a mission to find some epsom salts so that I could take a bath. The salts helped to dry out the ooze and I was desperate for some relief. They traversed through the city without any luck finally managing to secure some epsom salts from the spa at the hotel. I drew my first bath and spent over an hour trying to calm the raging skin. All of the tension, humiliation, pain and relief erupted and I cried and cried during the whole bath. I cried for all the time I had already spent and lost trying to get through this, I cried for the strain it had put on my family, and I cried out of shear hopelessness. But through my tears and the murky water filled with flaking skin, I also felt a sense of survival, of knowing that I would get through this. A sense of a deeper connection somehow, to myself and to those close to me.

Sydney and Andre were my rocks, my unwavering support system. Their understanding and care for me still tugs at my heart, and I was reminded of how lucky I was to have them in my life.

I saw improvements in my skin during the week and we made the best of the situation. My parents took things slow too, and we just let ourselves enjoy being together and experiencing wonderful new cultures. If anything, it meant our usual fast-paced, see-lots travel agenda was replaced by a more relaxed outlook that truly did feel more fulfilling. I think that trip is one of my most memorable and not for the obvious reasons of the difficult flare. I will remember it being a solid turning point in my journey where I really was at my most decrepit and lowest point, but that I still made it through. The support of my family was without a doubt, a huge contributing factor to that and I have come to realize and understand that finding support, from any-where and anyone, is a key fundamental to weathering the heartache and pain. But beyond that was the personal re-serves that I found. I never would have believed I would have been in that situation, but I did it. I pulled through. We have the ability to get through anything that pushes us down. The mental connection was pinging in my brain and I was really starting to get it.

Within a few months, that area healed. All that was left was some highly pigmented skin, but I was free and able to walk again and wear clothes. It was a marvellous feeling.

By the end of 2018, I felt as if I was finally through. That everything was on the upswing. My positivity remained through to 2019. My eczema and withdrawal weren't completely finished with me yet, as I still had flares, mostly on my neck and chest. But I had been through so much and seen so much healing that I didn't let the small stuff get me down.

Even though 2019 would be the most stressful year for me with other things going on in my life, my skin didn't go crazy, which I took as a good sign. I was still cautious, though, knowing that this condition can attack at any moment.

My neck was a constant sticking point. Perhaps it is where I hold all my tension, another reason why I had lost my voice and had the abscess in my throat. I would have little flares, then my neck would heal. I would experience some ooze and then deep wounds, but then they would heal a bit. I was frustrated with that a little but just soldiered on.

Throughout my entire journey, I had a constant worry about having an outbreak on my face. For most of my withdrawal, except for my neck, I was able to hide everything under clothing. My deep-seated embarrassment about my condition, something that had started in childhood, made me insecure about how I looked. With a clear face, I was able to still feel pretty, presentable, normal. I tried not to worry about it and just appreciated that my face was clear for the most part. I would obsess, though, and the very appearance of something on any part of my face, no matter how small, would cause me to have increased anxiety that was borderline irrational.

In January and February 2020, I had some trouble with my neck again. It seemed to be going through the ooze-flake-crust cycle but was definitely much more dry than anything else. I would go to bed and find a new flare somewhere on my neck and chest. I felt plunged back to the very beginning, where it was difficult to move, where I was uncomfortable in anything I wore. And then it happened. What I had been dreading for the entire process over the past four years. I had an outbreak on my face.

The one saving grace in this whole situation was now deteriorating into withdrawal and I couldn't stop it. All my worrying and stressing had made no difference. Topical steroid withdrawal had reminded me again that it answers to no one and has a timeline of its own.

I realized my immense vanity in the situation then, but I couldn't help it. I knew from previous experience that it would be only a matter of time before my skin would heal, but as I looked at myself in the mirror the situation felt dire. Unable to wear makeup and to put any cream on my face, I watched in horror as my skin swelled and crusted and flaked and aged. I had managed to get through the day-to-day before because I could hide my outbreaks under clothes. I could wear long sleeves and pants, cotton gloves, and socks. My face and neck could not be concealed, however, so every reflective surface I walked by showed me a person I didn't recognize. It was agonizing.

And then the world stopped and COVID changed everything.

To say that 2020 was a weird and strange year would not be descriptive enough. We all can remember the uncertainty, the isolation, the loss of touch and connection. For me, it felt normal. For better or worse, I had spent the previous four years unknowingly preparing for a global lockdown, which I was able to take in stride. For me, in some twisted way, it was a relief. While having a horrible time with my skin, I could hide the condition under a face mask and sunglasses. Going incognito was easy, and nobody even looked my way twice. For the first time in more than four years, I didn't feel like I was missing out on anything. I didn't have to make a choice, or be held back, because of my skin. Nothing in my day-to-day changed other than having Sydney home with me full-time, but I felt more calm than probably was normal. We all were mandated to stay home, stay inside, and limit contact with other people. Everyone was now in my boat, and my experience at the helm meant that I could keep my family afloat quite easily, and be there for my friends when they needed me. It was a bittersweet moment: a global pandemic that changed the world and humans forever was the one time I could finally heal in peace.

It was an odd place for me to be. People around the world were really suffering, mentally, financially, and health-wise. Countries were divided, approaches confusing, and protocols inconsistent. I wrestled often with my rather calm emotions in juxtaposition with a world in turmoil. My meditative practice helped me to realize that I can exist both in a world of compassion for others while not diminishing my own positive journey. That it is okay to be happy about something while others are not. One does not diminish the other.

That was one thing I struggled with for much of my life. When things were good for me, I felt guilty when they weren't for others. When someone else was suffering, it felt wrong for me to be joyful. Throughout my whole journey, I contemplated those thoughts, but it wasn't until the pandemic that everything started to fall into place for me. I realized that real change, transformational change, was not just the physical but what occurred in my spirit, my soul, because of the physical need. In order to move forward into a more joyous life, I needed to remember to continually live in control of my mind and thoughts. To remember that as the world turns and triumphs, falters and fails, I have to ride my own path throughout it all. I am in control of my life, my purpose only, not anyone else's. By healing and bringing that energy into the world, I help to contribute to the healing of the world. My physical existence is a visual reminder to me of what is going on inside. Yes, we can't ignore nutritional aspects of our physical existence, but our thoughts also help to manifest our physical, both positive and negative. I realized that my place in the world was small but significant. My reach was not deep, but it mattered. My priority is to heal myself. Heal physically, and most importantly heal spiritually. Connect spiritually. When I accomplish that, the vibration goes out into the world and helps support my family, and that exponentially goes out to touch others we come into contact with, and then who they come into contact with after that.

During the pandemic, it became crystal clear that we are all affected by and interconnected with each other. In small moments we can make changes to ourselves and our own bubble that, in turn, will positively affect someone else.

I was healing, yes—and happy about that, yes. I was loving my time at home with Sydney, finding new ways to connect with each other and new hobbies to explore. But being connected to what felt right to me is not something that I should feel guilty about. I realized that we all are here to feel that way. Our joy extrapolates out to bring others joy. I needed to remember that when you change your thoughts, you can change the outcome.

In truth, I was already starting—well, trying, really—to live my life that way. Over the course of my physical journey, I found myself going deeper and deeper inward to open up the way I thought and viewed myself. My therapy with Heather had helped to focus my energies more positively, but it also lit the spark that fuelled a desire to try to alter things for the better and ultimately for good.

On the outside, though, I *was* living a great life. In truth, if I hadn't decided to stop using steroid creams and just kept going on my mighty way, I would still be living well. Andre and I worked hard on our family, we all spent time together, we loved to travel and see musicals and experience things together. I never felt something was lacking in my life or that anything was disconnected. Yet I did have a general, vague sense of discontent. When everything was seemingly going great, why was I always wondering what more I should be doing? I couldn't relish or appreciate just where I was, I was always looking for more.

I found myself at a strange impasse in my healing journey. Dealing with the physical healing was all I had bargained for, but now I couldn't escape the reality that in order to find a state of permanent physical health, I needed to acknowledge and give space to how integral my own thoughts, beliefs, and ideas were linked to it.

I had no idea what all of that meant. I had no idea how to go about it. Whatever I thought I needed to do seemed to be instinctual only, as I had no strategy, no clear path, no idea about what all that meant. So to start, I just continued with my meditation and asked the question of where to begin. I continued seeing Heather and I dove into all those books I had so eagerly purchased. I tried to be open-minded and receptive to whatever I discovered, and I vowed that I would be honest with myself and not allow myself to make any excuses.

When I was struggling with my skin and looking for the answer to cure it for good. I never would have anticipated going on an emotional and spiritual journey. Quite frankly, it never even registered that that was something I needed to do. I had long ago accepted that we are all part of a larger Universal force and totally believed in everlasting spirit. I was an emotional person and I had a deep understanding of myself and why I felt certain things. Surely my physical journey to heal would happen regardless if I changed my state of mind (and to a certain extent I have found that to be true). What I started to discover was that physical healing can occur without additional effort. Eating right, resting, finding patience, enduring the pain: it would all lead to healing in the end. But there was a message in the troubles. I had ignored it many times before, believing that all the weird things happening to my body were just weird things happening to my body. There was no deeper connection other than pursuing a change in lifestyle or playing the waiting game to get through. That was what I had believed before, and to some extent the weird things resolved themselves.

But when one thing resolved and another appeared to take its place, it was becoming apparent to me that I needed to do more than just address each issue on a physical level only as I was never completely free from some sort of pain. Obviously, I had been missing a piece; there must be a connection between me, my spirit, my soul, and my health. The call had been put out to me many times. It was now time for me to answer.

Chapter 15

STARTING TO QUESTION

What did that mean exactly? At the time, it wasn't glaringly obvious to me that I needed to make some internal changes in order to fully heal the external. Some of the strategies I sought out to help with the pain I intended to use simply to calm my mind or ease some physical discomfort. In the beginning, that is all that my strategies really did.

My meditation helped to soothe my overactive mind and set my daily path as a less frantic one. The Epsom salt baths I took daily, often multiple times a day, helped to ease the constant pain my body was in during some of the more difficult stages. The CBD oil I used helped to steady my nerves and take the sting and zing out of the physical moments. I used visualization, breathing techniques, walking when I could, and sleep as actual physical ways to help with the pain. None of the things I tried were aimed at changing my way of thinking or to become introspective of myself.

I had one mission: get through the steroid withdrawal as best I could, use some strategies while I waited, and let everything play out.

Somewhere along the line, things began to shift for me. Subtle, barely perceptible, but little movements in the way I was thinking. Most significantly, as the months and years dragged on, I was left questioning what the real purpose of this journey was for me. When I thought back to when I stopped using steroids, I did just that, stopped using. I really didn't give it a second thought, it was an involuntary decision, almost as if it wasn't a choice. There was no ceremony about it, I just did it like it was the most natural and only path to take.

Throughout everything, I never wavered on that crucial decision. I never contemplated going back on the steroids, I didn't have moments of just throwing in the towel. As I became more disconnected from my body and watched it morph into something I didn't recognize, I became more steadfast in my resolve that this was the right thing to do. But why? Why was I so intuitively sure? Everything, every aspect of my life, was upended and suspended, with no guarantees or definitive timelines. There was no tried-and-true result for my condition, and I found that everyone who was going through it shared similarities even though every journey was unique. I would never have accepted that kind of ambiguity in anything else in my life, so why was I so eagerly allowing my body to go through such turmoil? How and why was I so sure?

There have been other moments in my life where I just did something, almost without thinking, because I just knew I had to. Going to school in France was one. Quitting my job was another. Regardless of the outcome or obstacle, I made the decision and felt instinctively that it was the right choice. Perhaps I was too much in my head with other things in my life at the time that I confused those choices with measured thought. Maybe in those decisions I didn't nurture or validate that it was a connection to my spirit that drove those directions.

Now, with only time on my hands and the solitude to think, I found my thoughts wandering and searching for some sort of clarification on what I was really going through.

But asking the questions and being open to the answers is not an easy task. The more I tried to look deeper into my life and the way in which I described myself, I wasn't overly jazzed by what I was bringing to the surface. I had read all the books and knew all the buzzwords. I had subscribed to the idea that you have to heal within to find true peace on a base level. I fanned that concept around like it was the golden ticket to happiness, but I didn't really accept or delve into what that concept really meant in actuality. It sounded good for everyone else, but as I was now faced with the reality of it being in front of me, it was a difficult challenge to step up to.

Maybe this is something we all face at one time or another. Maybe we are all given the opportunity to really take a look at our lives and make some changes that could only benefit us. Could other moments in my life where I was too busy to notice have been opportunities to change? Was that time of good luck or coincidence really a moment to give me pause to see how everything connects? How my thoughts and my outlook and the way that I view myself in my own life could directly affect the outcome of my day, my family, and my life?

I didn't have those questions in the beginning, just an ache in my being to know that I had to use this health crisis for something more than just pushing through an illness. I was feeling a need for profound change. Maybe because of the quieting of my world, I was finally able to hear this opportunity, despite the other ones I may have missed.

Chapter 16

TAKING A DEEPER LOOK

Looking deeper into myself didn't happen overnight. In fact, it was through the passing of time and the use of my other calming practices that my perspective began to shift. I started to take a look at my life—I mean, *really* look—and confirm that I owed it to myself to be honest and open to whatever I may discover.

I always knew I had shortcomings and behaviours that didn't suit me. While on the one hand I was wise and intuitive, on the other I was overly emotional and full of worry and anxiety. I was able to see and understand what my friends or family were feeling or going through and to offer advice or counsel. More often than not, I had it right. But for myself, I took a more critical eye. I could see the emotions behind what I was doing, I knew that the frenzy building up inside wasn't good, but I was incapable of changing it. I would berate and admonish myself for not being stronger and for not following the advice I would so eagerly bestow on others. I was a classic "do as I say, not as I do" kind of person.

And while I was aware that those emotional states of worry, stress, and anxiety did nothing to help my life or my journey here, I succumbed to their pulls time and again. I always knew I needed to change those thoughts and behaviours, but I never faced them head on or worked to move more fluidly through my life. I was stuck in a pattern of repeating behaviours and having thoughts that didn't serve me, but I was unable or unwilling to make the necessary changes to help myself.

Such was the case when I started my TSW journey. So much of what I had struggled with throughout my life crashed into my existence on the daily. My fits of hysteria and deep depression were necessary and warranted, but it never occurred to me that what I thought, or screamed, or did would have an impact on my healing and state of being. I just wasn't ready to help myself by listing the number of shortcomings I had and detailing how I was holding myself back because, well, I had enough to deal with at the time.

When I realized that my own personal journey to health wasn't going to offer any shortcuts, I started to think about treating myself with more kindness. I had pampered myself physically: taking baths, sleeping when I needed to, not taking on too much. But I still carried the same story about myself deep within me. I still looked at myself critically and would say things to myself that I would admonish anyone else for if they spoke about themselves with such negativity.

As I began to look at how my thoughts and deep held beliefs were tied to how my body performed and ultimately my true health, aspects of my personality or how I reacted to certain situations were coming to the forefront. I could no longer ignore the reality that a more fundamental change was needed.

What was most glaring to me were the labels I had attached to myself and the value I had placed on particular attributes and things in my life. For many years, possibly most of my life really, I had labelled myself as a high achiever and a go-getter. Carving out this part of my personality is not a negative thing; in fact, my need to achieve and advance propelled me to some great heights in my personal life and my early career. What was detrimental to me, however, was the value that I had placed on that label. I was worth more if I achieved and, more specifically, if I achieved some level of success in my career.

Those measurements or benchmarks for success were actually ambiguous even to me, but at some level I equated my value as a person with what I did for a living. I didn't know how to navigate around a conversation that usually started with "So, what do you do?" Early on in my life, I could easily talk about what I did, where I wanted to go, what my interests were. When I left the workforce, I was finding it increasingly difficult to shed the label of employment-associated worth from my thought patterns and vocabulary.

I had always liked to work, putting my full effort into whatever it was I was doing. Having employment was a privilege and working hard meant that I would see some reward, whether it be earning payment, gaining experience, or receiving enhanced knowledge. My parents were extremely hardworking people, and I witnessed very early on how commitment and tenacity could propel you to new levels. It was an up-and-up attitude, and I placed a lot of value on the concept.

What I was now starting to realize was that when I had pursued achievements earlier in my life, somewhere along the line I started to view them as measures of my success. Rather than achieve something solely for my self-interest and advancement, I began to tell myself that my true value lay in what I did. I believed others were judging me on where I was and what I had achieved. As I got older and my responsibilities changed, being valued for my hard work and my intellect became increasingly important to me. I didn't want to ever be spoken badly about. I wanted my colleagues and superiors to always be impressed with my work ethic and commitment. Who I was became linked to how worthy I was.

Of course, at the time I didn't recognize what I was doing. I thought I was just working hard, progressing, doing what is expected in life. But deep down, I was creating a seed of thought that only grew an unwarranted and untrue idea of who I was at the core. Instead of seeing my work ethic as a personal trait that would bolster anything I did, I placed the value on the job as the determinant of *my* value.

It was this running story of worthiness that needed to change. If I kept myself in the perpetual cycle of work equating worth and a career determining my value, then I would be constantly searching for and seeking out a reality that was impossible to maintain. Where along the line had

I lost the gumption to go for things because I knew I could? Where had I determined that without a real job, or the perception of a real job, I wasn't as worthy or carried less value? Could the story I had created in my mind be holding me back physically, and could the labels that I hadn't known I had applied to myself be doing irrefutable harm?

The short answer is yes. I know now that the way we speak to ourselves does an immeasurable amount of damage to our psyche and our bodies. The good news is that we can be in control of our self-talk, if we're willing to do the work. I hadn't realized how detrimental I was being to myself and that it was only me who could fix it. It didn't (and doesn't) matter what anyone else thought, said, or felt: the emotions of others really have no power over ourselves unless we let them.

I had created a falsehood, stemming mostly from my own fears and anxieties about who I was and how other people viewed me. Now, when I was at my lowest point physically, I was finally able to hear the wisdom that had been whispering to me for so long. The only thing that matters is what we tell ourselves.

Chapter 17

THE KID HAS SOMETHING TO REVEAL

As I mentioned, I know that the Universe gives us signs throughout our lives when we need to make some changes. Sometimes we can feel things deeply, a knowing that we must take one course of action over another. At those times, we are more in tune with our path and what our soul is asking of us. Other times—when life has muddled the message and we're overworked, overtired, or just not paying attention—we dismiss little moments that happen as odd or strange or "just coincidence" and so leave opportunities to change and improve unfulfilled. Plenty of times I brushed things under the table, unable to recognize them as signs to slow down or change direction. With many of the health issues I experienced prior to starting TSW, I was more concerned with stopping them than figuring out the deeper message behind their occurrence.

As I journeyed further into TSW, and as I looked deeper within myself, I realized that our bodies are wonderful litmus tests to how we're moving in our world and how aligned we are with our soul and ultimately our spirit. As I began asking questions, I was allowing myself the time and indulgence to hear what the answers might be. My decision to start topical steroid withdrawal was the catalyst to encourage a change in me that ran deeper than my appearance. It was a challenge to heal my whole body, from the inside out.

I needed a little help to get there, though—and it was my daughter who opened the door for me.

Our birthdays are one day apart. Sydney's is June 6, mine is June 7. While I had never really imagined myself as a mother, my daughter's arrival was one of the most important moments in my life. From the get-go we were connected, and having our birthdays so close means that the Gemini energy is really strong between us. I can understand her and feel her emotionally. As she grew up, this became a great asset to our relationship because I could put myself in her shoes and truly understand how she's feeling because I feel or have felt it too. The flipside to that, though, is that I found myself overdoing so many situations because our similarities could often lead us to an impasse.

I held on tight to Sydney and I expected a lot from her. As she grew, I wanted her to be respectful, polite, kind, well-behaved, and perfect in every way. I spent a lot of time talking with her, detailing how I wanted her to behave because at the time I thought I was preparing her for the world and doing my best to raise a well-rounded child. Andre and I were always on the same page about how to raise her, but while he was able to be succinct and to the point when disciplining her, I often couldn't let it go. She pushed my buttons, but only because I wanted her to be perfect. She was my best friend and we did everything together, but I was harsh on her if she didn't behave the way I wanted or say something the way I expected. I am a talker, and if she did something wrong, the art of cutting to the chase was not something in my arsenal. Quite, "to the point" was not my forte because I wanted her to *get* it. I would hammer home my argument, over and over again, just to make sure that she really understood what I expected and what she was to do next time. Subjects that my husband would be quick to speak to and then move on from would involve hours of me yelling, going over, rehashing even, while facing Sydney, who was in tears and clearly had already checked out. I felt compelled to drill things into her so that she really understood what I was saying, often believing that constant repetition would mean that the message would organically sink in.

I didn't like how I tended to go on and on, but I found it almost impossible to stop. The more I felt she didn't "get it," the more I harped on it. My parenting style started to emerge as a lecturer rather than a disciplinarian, and while I felt terrible and unfulfilled when things calmed down, I also felt incapable of controlling my diatribes. I didn't know how to manage myself and, honestly, I didn't know why I couldn't. Why was I so extremely emotional myself? Why couldn't I separate myself as a parent and act with maturity and decisiveness?

After spending some time asking myself those questions, I realized it was because I had never adequately prepared for, nor accepted, my role as a parent. And I let the long-standing story of career equating worth permeate my consciousness.

By the time I had Sydney, I had already been out of the traditional employment setting for a few years. At twenty-seven, I left my corporate event planning job to find something more. At the time, I was an emotional basket case, having nights with Andre where I was full of tears and lamenting how I needed to make a change. In actuality, I really liked my job and many of the people I worked with. But as the years went on, I felt myself shrinking in my role, becoming less creative and simply doing things just to get them done, regardless of whether I thought it was the best thing to do. I stopped fighting and was disappointed in myself for not staying truer to who I was. When the company underwent a major transition, I knew then that any change made would have to be from me. So Andre and I discussed what it would look like if I quit my job and we had to live off his salary for a bit. We realized that with some restraint, it was manageable and so one day in August I calmly resigned and started making plans for what was next.

This behaviour was completely out of character for me. I had never quit anything in my life, so it was a strange feeling to be doing something, really for the first time, that I didn't ask permission from anyone else. I felt it in my soul that it was a path I needed to take, and while it was difficult for me to turn and leave the colleagues and the position I liked, I couldn't comprehend continuing in the same way. It was time, even though I didn't know what was next.

That was the first time that I had to ask myself what I really wanted. Back then, as a newly married young couple, the world was for our taking. I didn't dive too deep into what my soul and spirit were telling me. I took the opportunity to jump into something completely different and opened a specialty dog boutique, fulfilling a dream of mine to own my own store and business. It was so fun and really allowed me to direct my own creativity and vision. The Pooch Boutique pushed me to work hard and directed me to tap into my confidence to do it all on my own. I learned about purchasing products, importing, and pricing. I used my creative skills to renovate the space with Andre, design the interior, and create my brand. I pushed my marketing skills to have the boutique be featured in our paper and on television three times. I was the store and it was me—and I felt proud of everything that I had created from the ground up.

I never told anyone that it didn't make any money. In fact, it took more than two years for the store to make enough to pay the debt I had incurred trying to get it up and running. I couldn't let on that it wasn't profitable or lucrative because that would admit my failure. I was so tied to the belief that what I did and produced was what made me worthy or successful. That label was so very entrenched that when Sydney was born and we decided to close the store permanently, I felt a reprieve that my new role as mom superseded any reality about the store.

So now I was a stay-at-home mom. This was not part of my life plan. I was supposed to be working, being independent, making decisions. While Andre built his career, made connections, and watched Leafs and Raptors games from corporate boxes, I was running around after my child, organizing appointments and counting down the hours until he got home.

I had spent much of the past ten to fifteen years cultivating an existence that my success and worth was measured by what I said I did for a living and now I was at home, attending to a baby, with no sense of value. While other mothers would relish in their new role, I felt unmoored and unable to accept that where I was was exactly where I needed to be. It wasn't that I didn't adore Sydney and feel immense love and joy being with her. It was that I wanted that in addition to a job that gave me an identity and purpose. I found it difficult to let go of one and jump wholeheartedly into the other.

This restlessness and uncertainty also caused some issues with Andre. We never argued much, but when we did, only one underlying issue was really at hand: my envy at his life. I saw him as breezing in and out, able to leave the hecticness of baby cries and diapers and exhaustion for adult banter and nights out for drinks. I would let this jealousy fester and then without warning, usually after a particularly trying day with Syd, I would explode. After hours of exhaustive yelling and sobbing, I would finally break down about not feeling fulfilled and longing for something more in my life than just toddler TV and stimulating extracurricular activities. Always supportive, Andre was open to me exploring whatever I wanted to do and would help in any way he could. But I couldn't really surrender completely to changing our family setup. I liked the role of martyr, playing the "look how much I've sacrificed" card whenever it suited me.

The strange thing was that I *liked* being home with Sydney. She was full of energy and tired me out thoroughly, but she was fun and happy and inquisitive. And she was so well behaved. She never had tantrums, and any discontent quickly subsided. Her first few months were challenging with colic and discomfort, but, really, from about six months on she was amazing. As a toddler she was interested in everything and so easy to be with. I always had to be on because there was no break with her, but "on" in the best possible way. To everyone she was the perfect child.

My irrational mind, though, still held strong to the belief that my worth was tied to a career. I just couldn't let go and it was affecting a lot of my life. For the few years before I started TSW, I would ride a roller coaster of emotions, unable to quantify why I was so envious of Andre and feeling strange that I loved being with Sydney on the one hand, yet feeling that it just wasn't enough on the other. I told the story that it was because I needed to feel stimulated and engaged, but really it was because I didn't feel important enough or worthy enough without a job title attached to my name. Who was I if I was *just* a mother?

About two years into topical steroid withdrawal, small mind shifts started happening for me. Faced with so much time on my hands and stripped of the freedom to do whatever I wanted, I had time to let those thoughts bubble to the surface with nowhere to hide and nothing to distract me from the truth. What was it that made me so unhappy about not having a job? Why did most of my arguments with Sydney and with Andre really revolve around that? When I was yelling at Sydney or arguing with Andre, why did I always end up saying I had nothing for me? Why was I so adamant about creating a role and title for myself that didn't just embrace where I was at that time? Why was I so insistent on casting aside my wonderful family and my role in it, to attach a meaningless label to feel value?

It took a lot more time for me to recognize, but the truth hit me one day, like a big neon sign flashing on. It was me. It was always me. Yes, I needed to parent Sydney and she did need to be disciplined at times. That's what parenting is. My need for her to be perfect, my inability to discipline without hours of rationalizing, and my anger at her when she did something wrong was magnified by my own insecurity. I realized that I viewed her as my job, and I always did things to the best of my ability and to a level of perfection. At some time, Sydney stopped being my daughter and started being the job I felt everyone judged me by. Her stumbles, and learning, and, well, her just being a kid were reflections of my abilities as a parent. The more applause and accolades she received were more acknowledgements of my achievements. She was good because of me. And when she wasn't good, it reflected on me.

It was my own self-sabotaging thoughts and ridiculous labels that caused me to be irrational in much of my approach with Syd. I equated working with worth. I equated a job with worth. So if I didn't go to an office or have a job with a title, then Sydney was going to be my job and I was going to make sure that job was done right.

And while this way of thinking meant that Sydney rarely got away with anything and developed into a polite and courteous kid, it meant that my nerves were almost always at the breaking point, and I was ready to pounce if she acted in a way that wasn't what I wanted.

My stronghold on her behaviour had its upticks. However, upon reflection now, it also created a confusing environment for her because she didn't know how to respond or how to act. When I got angry, nothing seemed to satisfy me. No explanation was quite right, and I prolonged my lectures just trying to prove a point. Sometimes, I wonder, if the point I was trying to make was really to myself.

As I began to settle into this new thought and gradually disentangle myself from the messy crosshairs of being a boss rather than a mom, I noticed small shifts in myself and in our relationship. I still maintained my expectations for her and still encouraged her to always try her best, but when she made a mistake I would usually address it succinctly and not carry on for hours, even after she apologized or understood the point. I didn't need to drill it into her because I began to see her again as her own person, not as an extension of me. It took the pressure off because I didn't need to control her, I just needed to help steer her. And it no doubt provided some relief for Sydney too. The frustration she must have felt at not being able to please me or act in the way I wanted must have been so difficult at times, so as I began to realize how I needed to change, I could see a general relaxing in her as well.

The same could be said about Andre. After almost fifteen years of being a stay-at-home mom, I was finally able to see his side of everything. The pressure he was under to provide for EVERYTHING: the house, cars, clothing, dinners out, trips, activities, appointments...

I never had to worry about any of it. And working in an industry where if you didn't get the deal done, you didn't get paid was incredibly difficult. My envy at him to be able to leave one life and lead another during the day was misguided and unfair. He needed to find the client, work with and negotiate the best deal for them, all while hoping that all this effort didn't result in them shopping his work around and closing somewhere else. He could put months of work into a relationship, only to see it not pan out, all without pay. Even though some of his after work events and dinners were sometimes work related, those times were needed to release the stress of his everyday.

I saw it now, much more clearly. When I let go of the fear of not having an identity, I realized that I'd had an identity the whole time. I was living a life that included rearing an amazing child, helping my husband build a business that supported us all, and being loved and supported by my parents no matter what I did. And I was happy. I had pushed so hard before because of my idea that a title or a position made me worthy and interesting. Instead of accepting what I really wanted and living for myself, I worried about what the world and others thought of me, and how they would describe me. It was a futile existence, ultimately never leading to any sort of satisfaction.

In my quiet moments when I shifted my thinking and dropped the labels, I felt calm. I asked myself what I really wanted and for the first time I stopped and listened. I allowed my spirit to guide me, my intuition to speak. I was right where I wanted to be.

This was heavy stuff for me and a huge breakthrough. For as long as I could remember, I had always had a goal and the goal was usually centred around pleasing others. If I accepted myself for what I was and accepted what I wanted to do and where I wanted to be, then pleasing others didn't exist anymore. It didn't matter what someone else thought of me because only I mattered.

I knew that this was only the first step, though, in my emotional growth and my journey toward living more joyously. And it wasn't easy. It was hard to look at myself and vocalize where I needed to improve, even if it was just to myself. It took days and months of small changes in my thought patterns to start becoming ingrained in my natural way of thinking. Daily reminders to let a grievance go, or focus my thoughts and energy on the accomplishments I had made, even ones that would seem insignificant, were important to help my mind navigate a new way of thinking and operating that didn't involve what someone else thought. Over thirty years of believing that you have to work hard at a job, advance, make more money, and sacrifice had to be rewired into thoughts of worth and value for me as a person, irrelevant of what I did for a living. I tried to acknowledge all that I had achieved so far in my skin journey, give credit to myself for the tenacity to stick to my path, feel good about the value that I brought to my relationships and family. I always had the insight and ability to acknowledge where others could change. I was an expert at giving advice, and I was usually right. It was near impossible for me to assess myself in the same way, though. But I did, slowly, and the improvements in my general mood and everyday life were measurable. I felt like I could cope better with setbacks with my skin or everyday disappointments. I was calmer, and able to take a step back and assess things with a clearer mind-frame and less anxiety.

It got me thinking a lot about what it means to live, really live, in a joyous and unapologetic way. I was finally able to see how the stories that we tell ourselves and the assumptions and projections that we put out there are the real hindrances to our success and happiness. It truly doesn't matter what anyone else says, or thinks, or comments on. It only matters what we believe and say about ourselves. I had heard it all before, but I didn't think it could be that simple or succinct. How we viewed ourselves was far more important and lucrative to our mental health, physical well-being, and overall joy than anything anyone else could project onto us. The mind, body, and soul are all connected, and without the full positive charge of one, the others suffer. But no one else can fill those charges, and no one else can deplete them. Our thoughts are our fuel. Shedding the outdated, untrue, and harmful narrative of ourselves allows our full being to run on all cylinders.

It's not easy, and it takes work, but I know first-hand how that work can pay off in the long run. It's not a simple fix, and reminding ourselves of our full worth, just as we are, is a constant loop that we must remember to tell ourselves, every day, until it becomes part of our being. The greatest gift we can give ourselves is to speak kindly to ourselves and nurture our thoughts, minds, and souls. It's a challenging but important key to finding and maintaining ultimate joy.

Chapter 18

IT'S A TOUGH ROAD, BUT THE TREAD GETS EASIER

Beginning to change my perspective on how I operated in the world was a pivotal step in starting to heal my mind and cultivate my spirit. But it soon became apparent that it was only the first movement toward a more complete shift in perspective—an inevitable progression for me to make.

As I started talking kindly to myself, more insecurities and fears bubbled to the surface. I tried to keep suppressing them, but they eventually began to boil over. Shedding the unrealistic labels I had placed on myself to determine my worth was only one facet of a complicated mind. I needed to unpack years of fabricated fears and anxieties and face them head on if I wanted to truly find balance in my life, where I would be able to maintain my physical health and feel uncluttered and clear in my mind. I had no idea that I would be heading down this path. While I had always tried to be honest with myself about emotions that I knew weren't good for me, I sometimes felt ill prepared to change them and learn how to live with less fear. Certain things in my life would send my body into waves of anxiety if I thought too much about them. Even though I knew that I was often letting my mind run away from me, I couldn't stop the train from accelerating.

Now that I had uncovered the path to not only more self-discovery but also committing to real change, I had to be brutally honest with myself and face those fears with the determination to think in a more healthy way.

One fear was that I would lose my looks for good. It sounds vain, and it is vain, but I put a lot of emphasis on how I looked. With my body in constant turmoil, I was okay if my arms or legs or other parts I could easily cover with clothes never fully recovered, but what if my face changed forever? What if I wasn't as pretty as I once was? What if, in my forties, I never looked like myself again?

It was illuminating for me to see how much I valued my appearance, or more specifically the attention my appearance received. On the surface I didn't think I was anything special, but when the second glances or compliments stopped, I felt so small. I was, *am*, embarrassed that subconsciously I felt this was. As my spirit kept trying to talk to me, I struggled intensely to break the thought that who I was was attached to what I looked like. I knew that my friends would still like me, my family would still love me, but would *I* still be able to love me no matter what the packaging looked like?

My other greatest fear revolved around money. Many of my disagreements with Andre or my need to work had lack of money as the underlying factor. Even as he and I worked together to build our life and family, I was never convinced that we were achieving anything financially. I always felt we were behind, lacked full financial autonomy, and that everything was on the brink of collapse at any time. It was not a rational way of thinking, especially since our equity and financial base continued to grow, but it was a fear that I was often incapable of shaking. I held on tight, would worry about being able to pay for things, and stressed internally when the bills came in. It was such a constant for me that I couldn't separate the fact that this worry and stress was not a part of me because it became a part of me, an adjective to describe me, just the way I was. But it wasn't healthy partly because it wasn't true and partly because it caused a lot of friction and discord in my life. As I faced this fear down, I could see just how wound up it was in my everyday thinking. I would always be running a tally in my head with how much things cost and whether I should spend or not. I would forgo buying something for myself, like a new shirt or pair of shoes, rationalizing that I didn't really need it and the money could be spent better somewhere else. I would often be caught in my constant loop of thoughts and unable to make a decision for fear that I would be spending too much and not saving enough. I would berate myself for certain spending I would tell myself was frivolous and unwarranted. Some would say that this was just prudent planning, but for me it was the fear of losing it all, that our unplanned and frivolous spending would push us into more debt and set us back in our financial position.

Before I started to really look at myself, I never would have defined these concerns as fears. Yes, I worried about how I looked and stressed about meeting financial obligations, but that was normal for everyone, right? To some degree yes, but that doesn't mean it's the way it is supposed to be. Just because it's common doesn't make it right. So tackling these thought patterns was difficult and challenging because I needed to reassess the story I had created about myself for most of my teenage and adult life.

Looking from an outside perspective and with an open mind, I can accurately say that my emphasis on my looks was obvious. Growing up with my skin condition meant that many times I was stared at when I was young and as a result felt ostracized. I was so embarrassed by feeling less worthy for so long that I felt gross or ugly when I was a young girl. As I grew into my teenage years, my skin flares became far less frequent so when I received positive attention for how I looked, I relished it. I so desperately wanted people to like me, so I often confused physical appreciation as acceptance. And because I participated in events that revolved around appearance—such as fashion shows, modelling, and some acting—I put a great importance on my looks. I realized that I had been traumatized by my skin when I was young. At a time when food allergies were not common and eczema was foreign to many people, I was different. I was the only one at my school who had issues with their skin beyond the normal typical problems like acne. I didn't have anyone to relate to. I didn't want people to notice me and so I became a shy kid, happy to sit on the sidelines, watching others take the lead, just glad to be included.

Looking back, I can see how I let my skin dictate who I was and what I did. Wanting to feel normal and just like everybody else permeated everything I did when I was in grade school and high school. When my skin improved, my natural being was allowed to come out a bit and I felt more confident and secure. But a piece of me always held on to the scared little girl who didn't want to be ostracized by her peers, and I worried constantly about fitting in and saying the right thing. I didn't value myself enough, again creating another story that equated my value with being pretty and thin. It was beyond societal demands and assumptions, as I didn't compare myself to unattainable images on TV or in films, magazines, and social media. The way I looked was the intrinsic value and worth I gave myself and was inter-twined and ingrained so deep in my psyche that I often couldn't and didn't separate it from actuality. I always com-pared myself to real people—the people in my life or those whom I interacted with daily—and used arbitrary and unrealistic benchmarks of what was attractive, acceptable, and liked. When I was described as intelligent, I felt good and strong. When I was described as also being attractive, that gave me value.

Some twenty years later as I sat in the crux of TSW, I was observing my body in decay and was disgusted with what I saw. I had replaced embarrassment with distaste, both thoughts feeding a narrative that was so the oppos-ite of confidence it was laughable. I was living a life that equated looking "perfect" to being worthy, or interesting, or liked. When I didn't like what I was looking at, I was really telling myself that I didn't like me. Instead of living in this body, nurturing it, talking kindly to it, accepting it, I was comparing its worth to a standard that I had created.

When I essentially lost my appearance, I had to find that spark of what actually made me who I was. I struggled for some time with coming to terms with the idea that Andre still loved me or found me attractive. Some days I looked so swollen, cracked, and bleeding that I didn't know how he could stand to look at me. So entrenched was my attachment to my physical appearance that I couldn't understand how or why he would still want to hold me or be seen with me in public. I was disgusted by what I saw, so how could he not be?

But this wasn't about him loving me through sickness and health. He didn't question things; it wasn't his view that needed changing. It was mine. And as one body part healed and another flared, I was continually reminded of how miraculous our bodies can be. As I allowed my body to shed and heal itself, I was scared and unsure, but I was also mesmerized. After an initial attempt to moisturize, I didn't put anything on my skin to help it heal or to move things along. My body cycled through torture and reprieve, pain and relief, all on its own. I started to create new ways to speak to myself. Faced with a shell I often didn't recognize, I re-evaluated what else I could bring to the table. All the aspects that made me who I was were not solely based on my physical appearance. I was a good listener, I was loyal, I loved my family, enjoyed playing piano, loved art. Everything that I really was had nothing to do with what I looked like.

The last part of my withdrawal was on my face, neck, and chest. Because these areas are usually exposed to the world, my acceptance of myself was really tested for many months. During this stage, I was the most exposed, unable to hide under clothing or through the trickery of makeup. It was the first time in most of my adult life that I had to be completely bare and natural. It was during this stage, though, that I think the most healing emotionally happened for me.

There was no escape: I didn't look good at all. It was my worst nightmare, a complete loss of anything I viewed as attractive. But as I took pause to sit in silence and accept what was, I became aware of what truly is. My physical body and how I presented myself to the world was important to me. And I accepted that I liked to look good and would always strive to put my best foot forward whenever I ventured into the world. But instead of garnering confidence from my appearance, I was harnessing the confidence from loving myself.

Other than my physical shell, nothing else changed during my withdrawal. I still loved the same things, I still thought the same things were funny, I still felt creative. I was me, a whole, not separate parts that came together. As I eased more and more into this way of thinking about myself, I felt lighter, more present in some ways. It sounds strange, even to me, but when I just accepted the way I looked at that particular moment, I felt relief. I didn't worry much about what other people thought about my appearance, I didn't shrink into oblivion.

I can't deny that I relished the day I would be free from the withdrawal and could wear makeup again and start to really work out. I didn't have intentions of not being proud of my appearance and trying to look my best. But it was no longer a benchmark that I used to determine if I was successful or worthy. I began to believe that it was an extension of who I was, not a reflection of what I was. Instead of doing things to achieve a certain benchmark, I now approached my health in a more holistic way. Instead of working out to be thinner, I worked out because it was kind and good for my body. Instead of berating myself for eating too much, or not eating the right things, I began to relax and just enjoy where I was that day. Instead of obsessing over blemished skin, I allowed my body the peace to heal in its own time. If anything, my physical healing from the topical steroid withdrawal showed me, with real evidence, that the body is a wonderful thing. It knows what to do when we let it do it unencumbered. My body and face and skin may change, but that was okay. I just needed to be patient and kind no matter where I was in my journey.

My relationship with money, however, was a much more difficult thought pattern to change. I've always had an interesting association with it. When I was growing up, my family would have been described by many people as affluent. And while that description is definitely overstated, I did have a very comfortable upbringing. To the outside world, my parents and I had everything: a nice house, lots of travelling, expensive cars. In reality, though, I lived in the crosshairs of what was perceived and what actually was. While my parents were, and are, extremely successful, an air of tension always surrounded our financial health. Regardless of how my friends and family viewed us, I knew that despite all the outward appearances of wealth, my parents were stressed just like everyone else and concerned about their financial stability just like everyone else. My dad's executive career allowed my parents to have incredible experiences, but they still had a large mortgage on the house and constant tensions with corporate change-overs. Both of my parents came from humble beginnings and endured financial upheaval and uncertainty when they were growing up. That uncertainty doesn't leave you, so when my parents started to achieve a certain level of success, it was difficult for my mom to surrender completely to that life. While my dad's position in business advanced, my mom would still worry about maintaining our lifestyle and making our mortgage payments. Even my parents themselves were a little at odds with how they viewed success and money. My dad believed he deserved what he achieved and loved to spend money on expensive things and enjoy the fruits of his labour. My mom was more practical and pragmatic and would be annoyed by some of my dad's extravagances. I was plopped right in the middle. I never had to worry about anything, but I could understand my mom's philosophy of being cautious. On the other hand, I appreciated that my dad spent for enjoyment. Both were extremely generous to others, always giving and helping if needed. They were especially generous to me.

For me, I saw money as a product of hard work and dedication, but I also feared not having it. I knew if I worked hard I would always make money, but how to grow it or how to maintain it always felt elusive. My dad was a brilliant guy, but he also built his career during a time when male confidence and arrogance were revered. It was a man's world, and my dad's ability to inspire dedication along with his knack for connecting with people made it a perfect time for his career. My mom was equally admired in her teaching profession, which unfortunately wasn't as financially lucrative as it should have been. My upbringing was extremely comfortable. I never felt spoiled and my parents certainly didn't shower me with expensive gifts, but I never wanted or needed for anything. There is a comfort in knowing that money isn't an issue, at least for the things that I aspired to do. I was so grateful for my family life, but as I grew into adulthood, I was seized by the fear that I would never be able to replicate the kind of success that my parents enjoyed. I told myself it was a different time and the possibilities that showed themselves in the 1980s weren't available to my generation. My parents were baby boomers living at the crossroads of opportunity and prosperity and that just wasn't what I was faced with. I set myself up to succeed less because it was easier to protect myself that way than believe I could achieve the same as my parents.

Now as I moved quietly alone in my home, I needed to unpack all my thoughts and fears around money and help my mind move in a different direction. All my obsessing and worrying about money didn't change anything in my life so, as I was starting to realize about a lot of things in my life, it was me who needed to change.

I had always held on pretty tight to money, likely because I'd spent much of my youth receiving the benefits that money can provide but all the while tense that they could end at any moment. Whenever I received my paycheque from a summer job, I would immediately put it into my bank account. It didn't matter what time of day it was: I made sure that once the cheque was in my hands, it was just as quickly deposited into the bank. I liked to have it safely secured, nicely tucked away, where I could watch it and manage it. That sense of control gave me a feeling of security. When I worked for myself, both during school and then after in my career, I didn't have a sense of dread and doom when I thought about money. Perhaps it was because I had a level of accountability for myself and I was in total control of my own finances. My feeling of security levelled any fears or anxiety I had around thoughts of money.

This push-and-pull worry I created about having and not having enough money was, I think, over-exaggerated in my mind. My relationship with money wouldn't allow me to see all the things I had achieved and been compensated for with money. The hard work and dedication I put into my summer jobs. The commitment I developed and displayed for my managers. The ideas and creativity that I brought to my work environment. I was unable to accept and tell myself that I was provided money for those contributions and that I would always be okay because I would always be able to provide a level of commitment and dedication to anything that I did. Money was very important to me, but my negative view on how to get it and how to maintain it meant that I was always feeling a lack, even when I was providing everything for myself.

Over the subsequent years, my anxiety about money, and not having enough of it, started to grow, almost irrationally and inconsistently. When I left my job, closed my store, and finally committed to being a stay-at-home mom, I relinquished most of my financial independence. As I helped Andre to grow his business and worked with him on building his career, I had to become more reliant on him and less on myself. It was difficult to rely solely on another person for my security. If Andre didn't work, we didn't make any money; his career in the mortgage industry meant that the steady income of a salaried job was no longer a reality for us.

How do you rely on someone else completely when you've been self-sufficient and independent for many years? That was what I had to unpack and tackle head on if I wanted to move forward positively.

Those were the moments when my financial fears would bubble over. The times when I felt out of control because I didn't have my own financial freedom. But it was more than that. Sure, having anxiety and fears surrounding the concept of money is not something I exclusively thought about; many people wrestle with that thought pattern. I coupled that fear with my self-induced story of self-worth being equated to a job outside of the home. In those moments I knew that I was thinking irrationally, that no one cared what I did, but I was incapable of accepting that. I categorized myself as being less interesting and giving less to the world when I didn't work or have a profession. I believed that if I didn't contribute financially to our family, I wasn't pulling my weight and I certainly didn't allow for the contributions that I made at home as brag-worthy or of much consequence. After all, my parents or Andre didn't go around telling people how great I was as a mother and housewife. I was a product of our societal belief that your answer to "What do you do for a living?" is the only measure of our success. And I fell for that thought hook, line, and sinker.

Throughout my time healing, it took years to come to grips with the fact that I was the perpetrator of these ideas. *I* was the instigator, the bully, the liar. Sure, these fears, anxieties, and worries are out there in the world and everyone at some time or another feels them, but that didn't mean I had to believe them. And not just believe them but actively live them.

I realized then that all of it, every bit of it, was not real. I knew this because no matter how much I worried about not having enough money, or not making my parents proud, or not having a career, it didn't change anything. Nothing. The stress, anxiety, and worthlessness did not make one significant improvement in my life at all. In fact, those thoughts just propelled me into continually thinking those same things, setting me on a hamster wheel to just go around and around the same issues. Now, as I was forced to be still and face everything I valued in life, I could honestly see that instead of preparing for the worst by thinking about all possibilities, I was inviting the worst scenarios in with every negative thought I had.

I was beginning to understand that my thoughts did matter. That if I wanted to achieve true success—whether that be financially or in health, or in any area of my life—I was the only one holding the key to open that door. What someone else thought about me, whether someone liked me or hated me, made absolutely no difference to the success I could have in my life. Only I held the power. By allowing negative thoughts and fears to enter into my consciousness, I was willingly handing over my power to be steered by an energy that didn't serve the best purpose for me.

I started to pay careful attention to my thoughts and the running commentary in my head. Every time a doubt or anxious thought entered, I made note of it and reminded myself to think more positively and to be kinder to myself. It is difficult to change a lifelong pattern, but it is possible and so, so important. Jealousy, stress, anxiety, one-upmanship, worry all originate from one central emotion: fear. Fear of not being good enough, fear of not being liked, fear of failure, fear of losing. "There is nothing to fear but fear itself." So simplistic in its design, but so powerful in its meaning. Fear is what stops us from living our full joy and finding our soul's true purpose. And it was true: all my fears were only hindering my capabilities, blocking the emergence of all my possibilities.

It still took time, though. Days and months, even years to train my mind to seek and answer to love and joy and positivity. With consistent practice and tenderness toward myself, I gradually began to trust in the power of positive thoughts and learn to banish my negative thoughts, fears, and worries. Now when a bill came, I would bless it and be thankful that I had the necessary funds to pay it. I looked at our mortgage payments and taxes as signs that we had achieved so much and were so fortunate to have a home that I felt safe and content in. As I practised this new way of thinking, I began to notice the fear and anxieties lessen and the constant restlessness and agitation slowly waning.

To say that I was shocked to be where I was would be an understatement. I had never anticipated that I would be overhauling so much about myself in my quest to heal my body. As each day passed, I found myself becoming more and more intrigued with and interested in connecting with my inner soul, and to figure out what I really wanted in life. I realized that the more often I chose to think and feel from a place of love, the more of what I wanted would materialize. The power to manifest was in my control, and that knowledge alone was showing me the way to take control of my life.

Chapter 19

OTHER THINGS MAY CHANGE TOO

I was now beginning to see noticeable differences in my life as I continued to challenge myself to be aware of what I was thinking and saying to myself. I knew that putting in the hard work would pay off in the end. I started to appreciate not only my body for what it was capable of doing but also what was more important to me. So far, all of my revelations were aimed at how I spoke to and thought about myself. It was inevitable really, that all of that work would reflect itself in the way that I interacted with other people and moved within the world around me. As I worked hard to value myself in a kinder and more honest way, I realized that I also needed to think about how I was allowing myself to be treated in the grander scope of things and what types of relationships I wanted to have in my life.

One of the values that I held deeply was loyalty. Well, if I'm being honest, I prided myself on having long friendships and relationships with people, regardless of whether they were truly supportive or even healthy. I wore it like a badge of honour, showing that I had friendships that lasted over decades, and I valued that consistency and commitment. During my self-discovery, however, I noticed that certain incompatibilities became more apparent and the cracks in relationships much more obvious to me. I had committed a lot of my time to some toxic relationships in my life. As I worked on thinking more positively, and approaching life in a less fearful way, those very relationships became more oppressive. Traits and qualities that were frustrating and emotionally draining before now felt even more harsh to me. Like when it's been dark inside and your first step out into the sun is a little blinding, I could feel the emotional toll more deeply now. I could feel it in my heart.

My pride in loyalty drove many of the relationships in my life from friends and family to acquaintances and colleagues. I had believed that if I put in the effort, worked and toiled to make those relationships last then it was a positive attribute that was to be revered. I had commitment, I was there for the long haul, look how special I am! Even when I felt depleted and drained from the toxic energy, I still pursued many relationships because I naively believed that my perseverance made me a better person. On the conscious level I wasn't looking to change anyone, but I was always hoping that the relationship could grow over time and change for the better. I was starting to allow myself to be more aware now that all of the effort that I prided myself for putting in, really was a futile pursuit.

Working on yourself can bring up a lot of things. Much of what I had believed about myself or carried as my identity just wasn't true, and while recognizing that and making efforts to be kinder to myself felt good and right, taking a hard look at my personal interactions and the other energies I allowed into my life was much more difficult to face. What was it about me that allowed negative people into my life, and not only allowed them in, but allowed them to stay?

In one word; fear. Fear at the prospect of not having these relationships in my life at all. When I had decades invested and long memories to draw on, my sense of obligation and fear of severing those relationships propelled me to constantly overlook things and push through. I was loyal after all. But it was becoming increasingly clear to me that in order to be emotionally and spiritually connected to myself, I needed to understand why I put so much effort into things that didn't really support the path I wanted and needed to take. I needed to evaluate which relationships would nurture my further growth and which ones would not. The important thing I kept reminding myself of was that all things in life, including relationships, take energy. If I was spending so much time and personal energy on healing my body and my emotional and spiritual well-being, then I could no longer afford to give away energy to something that drained me rather than lifted me up. My inner fears and self-sabotaging thoughts were all a massive draw on my energy; and if I was putting effort into turning that around, I also needed to look externally for what could be draining me further.

I also noticed that I wasn't alone in this at all. Almost everyone I knew was engaging in relationships that depleted them leaving them frustrated, overwhelmed and unappreciated. So many of us put effort into relationships at the expense of our own health and sanity and now I was in the position of questioning why I was and had been doing the same for many, many years.

It still doesn't make it easy, though. This wasn't about clearing house and saying, "Out with the old, in with the new." It was about taking a hard look at my life and all the stresses and the triggers for emotional upheaval and make a concerted effort to improve not only how I reacted to them all but how I actively engaged with them. It was difficult to stop giving in to those emotionally toxic and physically draining relationships. When you spend so much time working on normalizing actions and trying to make things work, it feels selfish to protect yourself and not give in. Like many people I knew, I was tied to a way of acting and reacting that, even though it wasn't supportive to my health, it was just how things were in my life. I was starting to see a pattern in how I interacted in many relationships and realizing that my need to please, to be liked or to not cause issues were often driving forces behind my continuing to push with certain relationships. Why did I feel the need to make things right, or keep things together if someone else didn't feel the same way? Fear.

But relationships are complicated, on so many levels that it is often difficult to extricate ourselves out of them, even when we know we should. Even when we are hurting or let down or emotionally depleted, we all come back, many times in misguided hope that things will change or, as was the case for me, not wanting to rock the boat and create more drama than I had to. How many times have all of us been there?

As I began to unravel my complicated feelings towards some people in my life I also had to be honest with myself on the role that I had played as well. In some cases, my guilt played a role, in others it was my desire of a particular outcome or connection. Maybe it was something in me that needed healing in order to close the door to the toxicity and negative energy that I was allowing from others to infiltrate in.

All of this was being thrust into my face because of my topical steroid withdrawal journey. It was really the first time in my life that I really needed support. My veil of personal togetherness throughout much of my life meant that I rarely relied on anyone else and almost certainly never asked for help or support. Throughout my life I had projected a persona of having everything under control, of perfection. I realize now, after beginning my journey and analyzing my actions, that I probably created the persona out of guilt from my condition and the toll it took on my parents. I didn't want to be reliant on anyone else, not just because of wanting to be self assured, but because I also didn't want to be a further burden. Even though I could feel emotions deeply and I could empathize and understand where people were coming from and what they may be feeling, my wall of confidence often blocked that from being seen by others or tapped into in my relationships.

As I was trying to change that within myself, I found that others didn't necessarily follow suit. This was surprising and a little upsetting to me. I thought that if I became more open, or allowed myself to be a little more vulnerable, then my relationships would only strengthen. In some cases, this was true and I found a much deeper connection to some of the people in my life that really has been a wonderful blessing. But for others, it just accentuated the cracks that had been patched over for years.

Some relationships with family, some with friends, even others that I thought were beginnings of more, became glaringly obvious to me were not helping to serve my higher purpose. They were toxic and unhealthy and most definitely needed to change.

In retrospect, I think that because I was changing my perspective, my energy and aura were changing too, which was likely the catalyst for the changes in some of my relationships. The negative energy from certain people just wasn't meshing with my new outlook. At the time, though, I couldn't understand why these relationships seemed to veer off course. Gradually I started to see that as my outlook changed, so did my acceptance of what I received in these relationships. Time was becoming very precious to me, and I didn't want to use any more energy on chasing down a friendship and trying to keep it mutually supportive all on my own. For the first time, I was willing to not force or control or push.

I began to release the feelings of obligation and guilt that attributed to much of my previous actions and control. I wasn't there to fix anyone, and I was happy to not expunge energy and time on a relationship in which the other party was not willing to accept an active role. And it was finally okay for me to let go and know that the

Universe will support the other person in ways I was unable to. I didn't have the desire to angrily shut my involvement in some relationships, rather, I wanted to change how I not only perceived them, but how I reacted to them. For the toxic ones, the ones that I felt entangled in the guilt and obligation, I allowed myself to breathe and shed the responsibility. For other relationships that I felt were often one sided, I gave myself the permission to put myself first and absolve the requirement to carry the relationship on my end alone. I still cared about these people, about what happened to them. I cared about their well being, health and stability. But now, I didn't take on the responsibility of making things right for them, of holding on to making memories because I thought it was the best thing to do. I had to accept that what I thought was best may not be appreciated by the other person, and no amount of involvement or hope could change how they interacted with me. It's okay to release and let go.

So, I just stopped. I didn't push for plans or try to force a situation. I didn't worry or fret about whether I was giving enough attention to a relationship and if they would still care about me. I took a step back and let things fall as they may. And, with some of those particularity trying relationships, I found that nothing really happened at all. The effort was not reciprocated and eventually the relationship dwindled and so too did my need to keep it alive.

When I stopped pushing and the others stopped trying, I felt like a weight had been lifted. I didn't feel alone, even though I had one less person to call. In fact, I realized just how draining some of the relationships were. As my confidence grew in accepting myself and appreciating myself more, my remaining friendships seemed to get better. I found that I was being more open and honest and in turn building deeper connections and friendships, even with those friends who I had many decades of time together. Without the clutter of trying to manage other relationships out of obligation, guilt, or fear, my energy was clear and space was made to enjoy my other relationships more and find those stronger, deeper connections.

With time, the sadness of the losses faded and any anger or resentment just wasn't there. I wasn't weighed down by pursuing something that was never going to be equal, and I was okay with that. As my body, mind, and spirit all healed, I was even more determined to have a life rich with friends and relationships who shared a mutual bond and support. I felt blessed with, and so much gratitude for, the friendships and relationships that were now blossoming.

This isn't to say that the ending of each of these relationships was shrouded in negativity. For many, coming to an end was simply the natural progression. But it was my lack of confidence and fear of change that prevented that ending from happening sooner. The transition was loving and caring not only for the other parties but mostly for myself. As I stepped into myself, the energy force shifted, bringing to light the incompatibility and darkness of some of my relationships. What potentially was always there now shone brighter for me to see, and my calmer perspective and shedding of labels and fears allowed me to allow these relationships to run their course. And that was the key: letting the relationship run its course. I wasn't looking to drop people from my life when we disagreed or things were a little tough. I knew which relationships were the real deal and which ones weren't supportive. Putting down the reins and relinquishing control allowed for a natural progression in which I didn't force or manipulate the outcome I wanted. I was sad when things ended, but it was a bittersweet moment as I cherished all the memories and turned to look toward a different future.

No relationship is a mistake. Every encounter, every friendship, every interaction has purpose and meaning. Most times, it's an opportunity to change ourselves and move our spirit and soul in a direction that enhances our growth. Due to our overactive ego, and all the fears we carry with us whether we're aware of them or not, we often continue some relationships for much longer than is needed for our soul to learn the lesson. When we are more open to our spiritual growth, we are able to see the friendships and relationships for the teachings and growth that they are there to provide to us. Even if a relationship was especially tough and was held on to for far too long, it too provides us with the opportunity to grow within ourselves and stretch our spirit even further to its purpose. I look back on some difficult relationships in my history and I can see how they helped me to develop resiliency and strength.

Change is good, and changes in relationships and friendships are natural steps in their evolution. Having the courage to move forward if something isn't right will always serve your higher purpose. We are not bound by whatever situation we are currently in. We are not destined to just accept the push-and-pull, the disappointments or upsets of relationships in our life. In fact, those relationships come into our lives to guide us to a better place to be. Take the lesson, bless the relationship, and gently release the grip on holding it tight. When we give room to breathe, we are allowing the energy to flow through and out of us.

I still have fond memories of those in my life whom I had to say goodbye to. I don't hold any resentment or animosity toward anyone. It was simply time. It was probably time a long time ago, but now I had the courage to accept the change. Life is richer for our experiences, and our friends and relationships help to build that fabric. And just like your favourite shirt or the one you've outgrown, it's okay to keep something forever while letting something else go.

Even more important though than closing a relationship is the ability to manage those that remain with calm and gratitude. There are some relationships that linger and ones that for whatever reason, we are not able to close the door to. Part of looking to discover ourselves is the ability to unlock the power to have control over our situations and manage our interactions with others so that we protect ourselves and block the continued transference of toxic energy from them to us. By valuing ourselves and and all that we have to offer, it becomes easier to manage the people who do nothing but drain us. When we shed our own negative labels and focus on centring through acceptance of our worth, we can assist ourselves to cope with the challenging relationships much better. So many times we all simply grit our teeth and bear through unnerving encounters with some family or friends. For me,

I would smile through all the negativity and then go over the injustices and irritations in my head for hours before and often days after. It wasn't healthy, and the "me before" knew that I shouldn't put so much energy and thought to a relationship in which the other party didn't see how their actions were affecting others, let alone be capable of changing their behaviour. My mind would run rampant though and I would wind myself up even before having to deal with these complicated people and situations.

Now I had a greater acceptance and understanding of what I valued in my life and what I was going to let in and affect me. By going within and strengthening my spirit, it was much easier for me to see the difficult situation for what it was—and it definitely had nothing to do with me. I realized that by facing problem relationships with an "I'm right, you're wrong" mentality, I was only perpetuating a tug-of-war in which I would never win. When I refocused the thought to one of more compassion and understanding, I shifted from "being in the right" to just being. What the other person said or did or how they acted had no bearing on the value and experience of my life. Only *my* thoughts and *my* actions were what were important to me. The veil lifted to show that the difficulty in the interactions was based in the other person's story. They were acting within the confines of the beliefs and labels that they had, many times, unknowingly placed on themselves.

So by removing myself from the equation and recognizing that the part I played could be interchanged with anyone, the relationship became less personal and direct. It allowed me to interact with more grace and less thought commitment. In all cases, it was about releasing control and just being, with nothing to prove and nothing to gain. When I started to view my difficult relationships in this way, it became easier to interact within them without it affecting all parts of me. Ultimately, I realized that with the relationships I was unable to break from, viewing them through the lens of love rather than being right made all the difference. Love for the other person, yes; but more than that, love for myself. If I had nothing to prove, no side to defend, and no agenda to push forward, then I was free from the entanglements of those difficult relationships. My body, my mind, and my spirit didn't need to have a reaction to how the other person acted or what the other person had to say. It was numbing, but in the most pleasant of ways.

When we make the effort to change ourselves, we must accept that some of the relationships in our life with change too. For some, the bond will only get better; for others, the cracks will show much deeper. It is imperative to remember that as we work to evolve ourselves and become more connected to who we are, we must release our fear and allow some relationships to take their course. With love and gratitude, we must move on from draining relationships to allow our spirit to grow more authentically. We can mourn the change and the loss but remain steadfast in the knowledge that we have gained and learned so much from the other person and it is now time to create new connections and relationships that can support a continued journey to optimal health—in mind, body, and spirit.

Chapter 20

SOMETIMES YOU JUST HAVE TO BELIEVE

As I began to apply the idea that much of my reality could be and was shaped by what I thought about myself and how I viewed myself in the world, I started to make more of a connection between my physical existence and my spiritual self. Meditating, correcting myself when I allowed negative self-talk to happen, and shedding the labels and untruths I had orchestrated about myself were all necessary and significant steps on the path to ultimate recovery. But the most important piece was slowly showing itself in everything I did. As time progressed, I felt more aligned in faith. In a faith that I would heal, in a faith that everything would be okay, in a faith that there was a true link between my physical body planted here on Earth and my spiritual existence.

I started to pray every day again. I used to pray when I was younger, and somewhere along the line—probably when life got busy, stressful, and messy—I didn't connect with that anymore. Now I was beginning to understand that prayer and faith together were just as important to my life as eating healthy food and hydrating my body. How could I possibly ignore the spiritual realm when I had a front-row seat to miracles happening? I believed that my decision to enter into topical steroid withdrawal had been divinely orchestrated. Something had pushed me to make that life-changing decision, and I'd been shown that if I trusted and believed, I would be following the path destined for me.

I could no longer ignore and separate my life on Earth from an eternal existence. A growing knowledge and love were building in me, and I allowed the belief I'd had when I was young to return. I think it was definitely an organic transition. Since faith and spirituality were concepts I used to subscribe to, my healing process only solidified these concepts into a deep belief, one that I couldn't ignore because I had witnessed it with my own eyes.

When times are tough and we're low or dealing with difficulties, finding faith, let alone keeping it, becomes a real challenge. During my most physically gruelling times, I felt that my faith in God or some sort of Universal existence waned. I yelled and screamed and cried at a God who I felt was abandoning me. I questioned whether God existed at all. It's difficult to have faith in something when you're in a situation that isn't seeming to improve. And it's especially hard to maintain faith when you feel that you've put your heart and soul into something, when you really try to get better, heal a relationship, overcome disease, and your progress is in a stalemate. How can you believe when everything is going wrong?

I asked myself that many times during my recovery. Why was I having a setback, why was everything taking so long, why wasn't it working?

At some point, probably after about two years or more into the process, I realized that I needed to pivot my thinking. I turned my attention to nature. By focusing on the fact that everything in nature knows what to do instinctively, I was able to ground myself for a bit and calm my existential questions. A tree knows how to grow from a seed into a sapling into a mature and magnificent sight. It understands that it needs time to be quiet in order to grow, so it stays dormant in winter, allowing its strength to build for growth in the spring. The same for the flowers and grass and every other living organism in nature. How are we any different?

What does this have to do with faith? When I stopped blaming God for my slow progress, I shifted focus to thank God for improvements. When I stopped seeing new flares as setbacks, regarding them instead as my "winters" to rest and heal, I started to have more faith in my recovery. In turn, my renewed sense of faith aided my ability to heal.

And so I prayed. I decided that no one was to blame for my situation. I was exactly where I was supposed to be. If I believed that moving into this journey in my life was divinely orchestrated, then I had to believe that I was trudging along the path to full recovery at the pace I was supposed to. I couldn't believe in one without having faith in God's support.

Faith for me is not religious. It doesn't seek a particular regime or ritual. It is simply a belief that you are here, in the position you are currently in, because you are supposed to be. And you will move in the direction you are supposed to when the time is right.

This was tricky for me because I was always moving forward. I found it difficult to be in the moment without thinking three steps ahead or focusing on what could or couldn't happen next week, next month, next year. I worried about the future, about what I would do, what would happen, where I would be. With a stronger reliance on faith, I was able to still set my goals, still have the desires and wants for my future, while finally being able to live right in the moment. Knowing that if you plan and strive, you will receive.

It was incredibly freeing to allow the mind to release the control and settle into a partnership and connection with the Universe. I could control the future, but not if I tried to manipulate it. What I thought and felt now would help to create the outcome I wanted later. I realized that my worry and tight hold on things that hadn't happened yet only increased the probability that I would strangle the positive outcome with my grip. If I allowed my faith to guide, then I was gently moving into the next moment, open to its possibilities rather than trying to force the outcome.

As I found myself in a new setback, I started to pray and elicit my faith even more. I had seen such miracles with my body before, so I knew they were possible. Holding on to the faith that I would continue to heal brought a sense of calm that I hadn't experienced before. As I watched the seasons change and saw the rebirth again, I began to see myself in the same way. All of us are the same way, really. Challenges are presented, we work through them, and if we have faith, we can then overcome them. Reminding ourselves of how far we've come by reflecting on where we were a year ago, five years ago, even ten years ago, proves that any situation we find ourselves in we can overcome. We can persevere. We can conquer.

I realized that this was perhaps the first time in my life that I truly believed in the power of faith. Maybe I had it before, long ago before the stresses and cracks of life beat it down into an unreachable concept rather than something I could actively ignite. Much like hope, faith was something that I told myself I had, but if I was being completely honest, I didn't actually believe in it.

Faith is a difficult concept. It asks us to believe in something we can't see, to hold on to a hope that we don't know is even real. Faith requires us to connect our ego mind with our spiritual being and trust that the Universe and God will support us. As I mentioned, I had been fairly religious growing up. My family attended mass each Sunday, I followed all the Catholic sacraments, I was dutiful and consistent and believed in God But I was now realizing that wasn't enough. Or rather, I needed to shift my focus from doing things to believing in things. I needed to hold, in my core, the faith that I am supported, I am loved, and I will heal. It takes time and commitment to place more weight into faith, but it's definitely worth it in the end.

As the years progressed and I eased more into this positive way of thinking, I realized that I wasn't looking to change myself or who I was or turn myself into some sort of meta-physical guru. I just wanted to be a *better* me. A more positive, happier, and optimistic me.

I started small, beginning with prayer, moving through to gratitude, and taking steps each day to talk to myself in a positive way. Every little step matters. Every little effort matters. Living with more faith and working to replace fears takes time and it isn't a race. Progress happens every day, in tiny ways. Over time, it starts to feel more natural to exist in a state that doesn't acknowledge fear but chooses to move in faith and optimism.

I no longer scream at a God who I feel has abandoned me, or question why I am experiencing where I am. I have faith in my journey. I have faith in my path. And most importantly, I am stepping out of my own way to allow faith to guide me along to my destination.

Chapter 21

WHEN YOU DIVE INTO FAITH, YOU CAN'T HELP BUT BE GRATEFUL

I have always been a glass-half-full type of person. Even though I was emotional and operated a lot in fear and worry, I was always hopeful for a new day, a fresh start, or an improvement in some way. When things got tough, I had a knowing in me that tomorrow was always another day. I felt grateful for what I had and my position in my life. I lived in a way that didn't knowingly take things for granted and I was always optimistic about what the future could hold.

That was before 2016. That was before topical steroid withdrawal.

As I've mentioned, there was a "me before" TSW and a "me after." This is true for all aspects of my life, including how I viewed and appreciated the people and things in my life and the experiences I'd had. Before, I knew I was lucky and felt gratitude for what I was able to experience: dinners, trips, concerts, the laughter of my friends, my home. Now, the "me after" realized that there was a meaningful difference between knowing I was fortunate and actively acknowledging it. Seeing the small, everyday wonders in our life and being truly grateful for everything that crosses our paths has immense value. I hadn't made that connection before. Yes, I was grateful for my home, and my car, for Andre's career and our health. But I was not seeing the value in everything else in my life that enriches it and deepens my connection to myself and everyone around me.

I began a gratitude journal, in which I challenged myself to write down ten things that I was grateful for each day. I wanted to know, if I forced myself to see the smaller things in life, whether my perspective would shift and I'd be able to feel more gratitude throughout my day and without prompting. Could I train my mind to view things with a less critical eye, and would this state of mind help elevate my mood and help me to move through each day lighter and more freely?

It was challenging at first, especially since I began this process during my struggles with TSW. Some days, it was easy to find gratitude. When my skin was in remission and I was able to live somewhat regularly, my mind could easily fill with things that I could give thanks for. On other days, when my mood was thick with frustration, or I felt depleted and down, it was more difficult to find ways to appreciate where I was and what I was currently enduring. I tried to persevere and, even on the dark days, force myself to be grateful for something, anything, no matter how small or insignificant it may have seemed.

I would write my gratitudes in my journal and read them to myself throughout the day. Some days I was grateful for the big things: having a home to live in and protect me, enjoying the comfort of my air-conditioned car, savouring the wonderful dinners at our favourite restaurants. But, over time, as I pushed on, I started to see the beauty in the small stuff. I began writing down all the less obvious things. I was grateful for the sun on a warm day, thankful that I could take my dog for a walk. I was grateful to be able to help Sydney with her homework, or that Andre was managing okay at work. I was grateful for my bed, which helped me heal and provided comfort for me during the darker times. I realized that the very act of acknowledging ALL the wonderful things in my life, no matter how little or insignificant they may seem, is what elevates each one of them to a higher meaning and purpose. The more I gave thanks and was grateful for these small conveniences and luxuries, the more I began to appreciate everything that I had and was experiencing. And then something really interesting happened. My appreciation for all the little things actually helped to make me more content with where I was in my life and with all that I had. Yes, I still dreamed about vacations, or thought about upgrading my home, but the urgency or need simply wasn't there anymore.

As an example, my husband and I really loved our home, but for about four or five years we were actively looking to move. We would inspect our house critically, finding things that weren't perfect, which would set us on our quest to fulfill all our needs in a new home. Sometimes we felt that our neighbourhood was getting too busy; other times we thought that maybe a house in another area would appreciate more and be a better investment. We longed to finish our basement but felt it may be easier if we just found a house with that already done. We even dreamed about something as silly as wanting new flooring or having a better bathroom. My home was wonderful, but I have to admit: I didn't put my whole love into it because I was often thinking something better was out there. I had a restlessness about me, a yearning for something that I thought would finally be everything that I, and we as a family, would need.

My recovery helped to change that. More specifically, my focus on gratitude helped to solidify my acceptance of my home's true value. I was thankful that I had the space to move around while I spent days and months confined to the house. I was grateful that I had a beautifully big bathtub where I could take soothing baths. I was grateful for the privacy we enjoyed in our backyard. Each day I noticed more of the positives in my home rather than the things that needed fixing or could be found somewhere else. My home provided comfort, privacy, protection, quiet, convenience, and light. All of that far outweighed anything else.

Gratitude didn't mean I just stopped dreaming or striving for something different or better. I will always be open to moving and interested in real estate. It's a passion of mine. But having more gratitude for the things I *did* have meant that when the time is right for a change to happen, it would happen. Gratitude opened the door to allowing what can be to potentially be. By focusing on the positives and my abundance, I shifted the energy and ultimately helped to create even more to be grateful for.

This quickly became a daily practice, something that I just did, and soon it felt natural and right to give thanks for all the wonderful things I could enjoy. More importantly, though, it felt good. I like to start my day with my morning prayers and then a list of what I am grateful for. Some days I am grateful to be able to get out the house; other days I'm grateful that the sun is out and brightening the day. By starting with a positive note, I send out the intention that all is okay in the world. I jumpstart my emotions to skew on the positive side, and it sets up my whole day to operate from that mind frame. And again, it just feels good.

Many days, the "me before" would wake up and dread the day ahead. I was so trapped in my limiting thinking that I could only anticipate how difficult the day would be navigating it in my body. The turmoil that I felt often clouded my perspective and I approached each day just trying to get through it. As I practised more and as time carried on, I couldn't really be in a bad mood, even if I tried. The optimism that gratitude gives is unmistakable. Even if I was feeling down or tired or not really grateful at all, I still made myself to pray and give gratitude for something, anything, and it always shifted the focus of my outlook.

My glass-half-full perspective took on a new meaning, even during troubling days. Each day is ours to choose how we want to see it and how we want to live it. The one guarantee we have, exclusive to ourselves, is domain over the direction our day will take. Faced with challenges and tragedies, it is our choice alone in how we want to see them and react to them. No matter what, there is always something to be grateful for. If we can find that kernel, that one thing that reminds us there is good, then life is inherently enriched.

Chapter 22

CAN MY THOUGHTS REALLY CREATE MY REALITY?

I found myself spending a lot of time reading books about how what you think can help shape your reality. Initially I gravitated toward these publications as beacons of hope as I sailed unanchored through those confusing first months and years. They offered some level of hope, even if I didn't commit fully to their message. As time wore on and I became aware of my need to rethink how I was approaching my daily life, I returned to these books with a fresh eye and open mind to read what they were *really* saying.

Could I relate to the idea that any ailment could be caused by the thoughts we have? Could someone's cancer diagnosis be attributed to deep-seated thoughts about control and long-held hurt? Could another's heart disease be a result of ongoing negative thoughts embedded in the subconscious? Could my recurring eczema be due to not only topical steroid addiction but also the negative thought patterns that had plagued me growing up?

I don't know. It's fanciful and hopeful to pass the buck to mind over matter, but is it realistic? Why has rampant disease in our culture increased only because of lifestyle choices and poor self-care, or so we believe? Can you really cure yourself by changing the way you think?

I'm not a doctor nor a historian, so access to historical data or scientific studies about this concept was not readily available to me. It didn't really matter, though. What mattered was whether I was willing to be open-minded enough to read through these books again and heed their messages. I had already been working on how I viewed myself within the context of value and worth, so wasn't how I spoke to myself in the little moments an equally important step in my journey? And wasn't it logical to say that letting go of anger, animosity, and resentment went hand in hand, really, with a better, more optimistic, and healthy view of life?

When I first bought these books, it was in the initial stages of my ordeal so I was getting my hands on anything I could. I was desperate, hoping that I would find something within this multitude of pages that would shine a soft light telling me to hold on. I read ferociously then, finishing one book and immediately picking up another as my mind searched each chapter for clarity. And I did find great comfort in those first read-throughs. I found peace in the calming tone and small sparks of hope. Even if my thoughts were not fully aligned for health, I received the feeling that I was loved and supported by the Universe. Although these books gave me a spiritual connection, those first few years I didn't really feel it, or maybe I didn't have the ability to dive deeper into myself and change what was brewing within. The writings helped steer me to reconnect with my spiritual side and think more about God and my alignment to Source. At the time, that was the message I needed in my recovery. Now I was in a position to be more receptive to the teachings that many of the authors proclaimed. That beyond prayer and connection to the Divine, part of my reality is shaped by me. I have a hand in my journey, and the trajectory of what I can do is ultimately controlled by what I am willing to let go of mentally and replace with positive thought patterns.

There are countless books available that touch on the connection between mind, body, and spirit and all of them generally have the same tenet at the core: you are what you think. It's a simplistic message, but one that conveys the ultimate truth. Our thoughts have a huge impact on our health and well-being, and if we want to have sustained health, we must manage how we speak to ourselves and the level of negativity we let fester in our bodies.

As I read my old favourites again, I found new books and studies that further solidified the concept for me. Stories of people with a terminal illness who changed their lives and thoughts and saw the illness dissipate and, in some cases, completely disappear. More and more accounts of mind over matter were appearing to me, and I couldn't deny the strong connection that has been proven between the state of your health and the state of your mind.

I liked this idea a lot. Getting through a physical illness is one thing, but ensuring that you can maintain optimal health is another. While I was "all in" for lifestyle changes like diet, exercise, sleep, and stress reduction to help heal my body, I couldn't deny that only doing those things wouldn't set me up for true health. I had to accept that my thoughts and my mind played a huge role in how my body reacted. I couldn't guarantee that I would always be one hundred percent healthy, and I couldn't see what the future had in store for me, but I was now determined to do the best that I could to create the optimal environment for long-term success.

It's easy to get into, and remain in, a pattern of self-loathing. It's the small moments that pile on to each other and start to pick away at your well-being and health. Short thoughts of not being good enough, or passing moments of feeling inferior. Worry and stress are sneaky bedfellows who gnaw away silently, creating a space that's ripe for disease and illness.

However, as easy as it is to fall into those thought patterns, it's just as difficult to get out of them. But difficult doesn't mean impossible. Slight changes can over time become big amazing changes and the benefits are immeasurable. So, I started small.

Each time I would catch myself thinking something negative about myself or the situation I was in, I would gently support myself to change the meaning behind those thoughts. I didn't force myself to be perfect right away, nor set the unrealistic expectation of banishing all negativity. These thoughts are insidious, creeping in through an unguarded gate. Berating myself for not doing better, or for letting myself slip into old patterns, would do nothing to shift the focus and intention. Kindness and patience were all that were needed.

I began to create mantras to help set the tone and inclination for the day. I would repeat them over and over again to help kickstart my brain into thinking more positively. Whenever I would sense my thoughts veering in a negative direction, I would remind myself how far I'd already come. It was helpful to write the mantras down and have them available, depending on where my thoughts were on any given day. For me, thoughts of regret, remorse, hopelessness, and fear popped most often into my head. So I created mantras that helped me address those feelings and retrain my mind to think and feel more positive about them.

I am perfect health.
I am eczema free.
I am prosperous
I love and am loved.
I have perfect skin and I am vibrant.
I am that I am.
You are working so hard.
Every day is closer to your goal.
I am life.

There were many more along the way, but each mantra helped me focus on what was right with me and with my life rather than what I perceived was wrong with me or with what I was doing. Eventually, over time, I didn't need as many intentional reminders to shift into positive thinking.

It started to become more natural for me to quickly correct myself when I was moving toward a darker path. The fleeting thoughts that *maybe it wouldn't be okay* and *I would never be normal again* did try to creep in, but I had trained my brain to see the upside first so those thoughts never really stuck.

Your mantras will be different than mine. Your path will be different from those of everyone else. There is no right way or wrong way. There is only one way: what feels right to you.

Can I say for sure that by changing my thoughts, I changed my health? Honestly, no, I can't say with certainty. When I was in the depths of my recovery, everything I tried and committed to was like a life preserver pulling me through the watery depths that were too dark and murky to navigate alone. They helped me endure. I was healing my body from decades of abuse that wasn't totally a result of my thoughts or my lifestyle but rather a chemical. What I can say, without a doubt, is that by changing my thoughts and ways of thinking, I am supporting my body and my mind into a healthy state from this moment on. By pushing the doubts and worrisome thoughts to the side, I am allowing for a more positive equilibrium in my body that can do nothing but contribute to my well-being.

One thing I do know for certain is that, if anything, working hard on changing our thoughts will ultimately help to change and alter our view of ourselves, our lives, and our abilities. And that is truly the ultimate success.

Chapter 23

THE UNIVERSE HAS MY BACK

As I learned these new lessons about myself and new ways to approach life, my actual life continued to carry on. I still found myself enduring the up-and-down swings of my recovery, but experiencing longer periods of remission in which I could embrace a bit of normalcy here and there. It was so freeing to walk without pain and so exhilarating to be able to wear short sleeves again. In those snippets of time, what I noticed most was that while I wasn't fully able to believe that I was out of the woods, I felt a growing appreciation for all the little things in life. Everything I had taken for granted now seemed so amazing and glorious, probably because it had all become so fleeting for me. Going for walks, enjoying the warmth of the sun, working out, cooking dinner: each one meant more to me than I thought I could or would ever need to experience.

I also felt calmer. I still had outbursts, I still became angry and fearful and confused, but it was easier to manage those emotions and not lean into them. Perhaps it was because I now realized that no matter what I felt, it wouldn't change my position with my health—only time could do that. But I hoped it was deeper than that: that all the work I'd been doing to change my perspective was actually taking hold and creating some real change. It felt positive and good.

I started to see some real results in how I handled the day-to-day aspects of my life. Through meditation, the releasing of labels, and working on my positive thoughts, I was noticing that my reactions were changing. Even though I found moments of reprieve with my body and my skin, it continued to be a roller coaster ride of uncertainty and pain. One day was amazing, only to be followed by an unexplained flare. The unpredictability of it all humbled me to let go of expectations and focus on how to deal with challenges as they arose. My skin was the one thing that I literally couldn't control, and it taught me a good lesson in letting go and surrendering to what will be. I had never given in fully to the idea that the Universe had a plan for me and that I was and would be supported in everything I did. On some level, my spirituality was strong; but on another deeper level, I felt that what I did with my life really determined my reality. To some extent, that is true. We have to be active participants in our own lives and destiny, but I was starting to awaken to the concept that if I let go, stopped holding on so tight, life could unfold in better ways.

And the Universe sure had plans to solidify that concept for me.

After Andre and I were married, we got a dog named Maxwell, a lively and cute Havanese. We navigated parenting our puppy as newlyweds, figuring out how to take care of this other living thing. We both had had dogs growing up, but it was a challenge for us to balance our social independence with being there to train and nurture Maxwell. We were young and admittedly made mistakes in our training, but we loved him and he held a piece of our heart.

When I operated the specialty dog boutique, I took Maxwell to work with me every day. With long hauls of silence between customers, he and I soon bonded, becoming close companions. I would put him in his fashionable coat and booties for our walks. This was at a time just on the cusp of the trend to pamper dogs with clothing so everywhere we went Max got attention for his stylish clothes and his ability to keep his boots on. But for all his cuteness, he was a tricky dog. While he was so much fun and quiet at home, he became a barking terror on walks. He would bark furiously and ferociously at any dog he would see, scaring everyone around us. Endless training didn't seem to do the trick, so Andre and I learned to constantly be aware of who was approaching us, then crossing the street well in advance of any interaction. Max was also very agitated, licking himself constantly, and no attempt at soothing him made any difference. He would pee on visitors, try to bite their clothing, and would hump at random. We tried three or four different trainers and training methods, sticking to them studiously, but nothing seemed to work. We accepted that he would just be an at-home family dog and that interacting with other dogs or accompanying us on outings wasn't in the cards.

When Sydney was born, Max was curious and gentle with her but ultimately a little jealous. While we tended to her, he would pee and poo around the house to assert his dominance. My day was filled with taking care of an infant while chasing Max around, making sure he behaved himself. But we accepted Max for who he was and modified out lives accordingly. We fell into our rhythm as a family.

It was a strain, though. I know that some would find it ridiculous that I was stressed about my dog, but in a home where I valued quiet and peace he tore that concept apart. Plus, I was so frustrated that through all my effort, I just couldn't make much headway with him. It was embarrassing at times and stressful when we left him with people if we went away. My parents were great about looking after him when we needed them to, but I know they were just gritting their teeth, trying to help us out rather than really enjoying him at all.

For all his challenges, he was fun and gentle and playful. We had fun within our walls and Sydney loved him a lot. Over the years, he started to have a few health issues, but he also mellowed out and became a really joyful dog to have around.

He also became my biggest supporter.

When I first started my TSW journey, Max was about twelve years old. He had started to go blind, but it didn't really affect his everyday living. The first year for me was rough; I was in a lot of pain and really confused. I cried a lot. Maxwell was there, though, comforting me and staying by me. He helped me find a strength to get through the day when it felt at times that I couldn't go on. He'd kiss me and cuddle me and look at me with compassionate eyes. We bonded even more than I thought possible.

The next few years we saw Max's health deteriorate. We almost lost him through a bout of pancreatitis, but with emergency care he pulled through. He became totally blind, and dementia soon set in. He was unable to walk up and down stairs, so we needed to carry him every time. He would stare for hours at corners of the room, unable to orientate himself, and he cried constantly through the night. By now, he was sixteen and in rough shape. Despite all our trials together because of his stressful behaviour, we understood each other, and his unwavering support of me through the day-to-day, when it was just us in the house together, created an incredible bond that was heart-wrenching for me to contemplate losing. He was fading, but I didn't want to let him go. It took Andre and I about a year after Max's pancreatitis to realize that it was cruel for me to want him here for my own selfish reasons. With weary broken hearts, we agreed it was his time to go.

I took it hard. It surprised me that I'd become so attached to a dog that had created so much turmoil and stirred up such emotion in my life. I hadn't felt the bond that many owners feel with their animals—their pets become part of the family, going everywhere with them—until much later in Maxwell s life. But our bond was so strong from those horrible years for me that I grieved him for a long time. After about six months, Sydney started asking about when we could get another dog. Andre was open to it, but I was adamantly against it. Even though Max had eventually calmed down and we had some great times together, the stress of even thinking about possibly going through what we did with him ended the discussion for me. I had freedom now. I didn't worry about getting home for the dog or having to care for an animal that couldn't go up and down the stairs on its own. It was selfish, but I was appreciative of the rest. I was pretty resolute that our dog ownership days were over for some time.

As we rolled into 2019, Andre and I had endured some really challenging times, both with my skin and one of the worst flares I'd ever had as well as personal family difficulties and issues relating to his work environment. We were optimistic as the year started, though, and I felt that I was in a new headspace, calmer and more grounded, as I'd had more time to develop my meditation and positive thinking approach. Still, I was certain that we wouldn't be getting another dog, even as Sydney's weekly probing continued.

It was sometime around March or April that I found myself at lunch with the two of them, chatting about stuff when the conversation turned to dogs again. This time, I didn't shut Sydney down right away; in fact, I found myself scrolling through the Internet on my phone, looking for information—on what, I wasn't so sure. I landed on a Kijiji ad for a bich-poo puppy and inexplicably found myself turning my phone to the two of them. "Isn't he cute," I exclaimed. Sydney's eyes lit up and an excited tension started to build. Like them, I was in massive disbelief at what was happening. What was I doing? What had come over me? In the short time span of about thirty minutes, we had gone from casually talking about puppies to me calling the number in the ad to inquire for more details.

This was insane, and definitely not something I usually did. I was researched, planned, intentional. I was not impulsive, spontaneous, or carefree with decisions like this. It was as if an unknown force was guiding my hand and encouraging me to keep moving forward. Even though this was totally against my nature, I didn't feel out of control. It felt, strangely, right.

Perhaps the weirdest of all was that I found myself mere hours later meeting up with a woman in a Tim Hortons parking lot to look at two puppies in the backseat of her car. It felt like a clandestine deal shaking down but also felt so right. My year-long stance on a dog-free life had swiftly been axed in one day. We selected the puppy we wanted and agreed to pick him up in a couple of weeks.

This was new territory for me. The "me before" would have worked out every scenario, fretted over training and the dog's personality, worried about sleeping and puppy issues—all before even committing to a dog. Now the "me after" was excited about the possibility, with no thoughts about issues or troubles or difficulties. It was as if my go-to way of being had been replaced by a more normal, calmer version of myself. Was this the result of the work I had done internally, of trusting that things were unfolding as they should be?

That's how I knew the Universe had a plan for me. Against all odds and attitudes, we were getting a puppy— and it seemed like I was the leader in making it happen.

The next few weeks passed quickly, and it was time to pick up our little guy. We had shopped and outfitted our home to welcome him with all the comforts. The moment

I held Bentley, I fell in love. It was like he was destined for us, meant to join our family. He was so cute, so lovable, so loving.

And then I got Bentley home and all the old insecurities came bubbling up. I was with him throughout the day when Andre was at work and Sydney was at school. While they both took on the challenge of training him, the bulk of the work was in my hands. And I was failing miserably. All my past stresses from Maxwell emerged, and I found it draining and distressing trying to train Bentley. Everything he did, I perceived as wrong, and I was yelling at and reprimanding him more than encouraging him. The "before me"—the one who wanted everything in perfect order, who yearned for structure and consistency, who hated mess or things in disarray—was driving me, and I was losing it.

In a moment of weakness, I broke down and told Andre I couldn't handle it and maybe we should find Bentley a new home. I was so stressed out that I was willing to re-home him, something I ordinarily would find abhorrent. But I decided to give it one last shot and brought in a trainer . Known for his skill in getting puppies and dogs to respect their family members and helping the humans to train a happy and healthy dog, he worked with me to refocus Bentley and train him properly from the beginning. As Bentley and I worked together, I started to see everything differently. Bentley was a member of our family and just a puppy. It was our job to make him feel love and to let him know the ground rules. In my panic of thinking of him potentially ruining the calm I craved, I missed the point that showing him the best way to behave in our family may be challenging but it didn't have to be hard. It wasn't him, it was me. I was projecting all my worries and stresses onto him. I didn't need to change anything I was doing in training him, but I did need to alter my perception of what was acceptable. Bentley wasn't Maxwell, and I wasn't the same person who had neurotically tried to train my previous dog. I had a new perspective and appreciation now, and I needed to remember to tap into the joyfulness and lightness that can occur when you loosen the reins and relinquish control.

From that moment on, Bentley has been a joyous addition to our family. He's friendly, great in the car, playful, and, best of all, loves to snuggle. While Maxwell taught me about commitment and unconditional love, Bentley continues to teach me that life is about living in all the moments. He has reinforced for me the freedom in letting go of the little things. He has also taught me about letting go of the past, of what used to be, of what was. Bentley has his own personality, his own gifts, his own soul. By connecting with him beyond the owner-dog dynamic and viewing him as an integral part of our family, I have been able to see all the little mishaps as just the little things in life. His muddy paws on the floor, oopsy accidents, toy stuffing all over the house… those are all fun, clumsy, exasperating parts of life. But they're the good stuff too.

It's funny yet interesting that it took a cuddly ten-pound little guy to show me just how disconnected I was with what really mattered. I saw, quite blazingly, how my need to control and my desire for everything to be in perfect order was causing undue stress in my life. How some of the values I was holding, and considered necessary, actually weren't all that important.

Bentley joining our family came at the most perfect time. The remainder of 2019 was very difficult for us, with the death of my dad and Andre leaving his business partnership and starting anew. We were challenged and nervous, sad and scared, but Bentley was the constant joy, reminding us to push forward and seek happiness each day. He was the ultimate comfort, something we didn't realize we would need until we did. But the Universe knew, and I will never doubt again.

Chapter 24

IS IT A WHOLE NEW ME?

I continued to marvel at how my life was turning out. For someone who was the consummate planner, I hadn't planned or tried to orchestrate any of the things I found myself involved in. I still couldn't believe the direction I was now in, where my physical healing was seeming to take a back seat to my mental stability and overall outlook. How did a quest to heal my body lead me to completely overhaul everything I said to myself and thought about my life?

The only answer I could find was that I was exactly where I was supposed to be. My only sadness was that I didn't see it clearly enough before and that I needed the nudge from the Universe to begin the work on myself . Perhaps I was still so closed off to the idea of internal healing and rebuilding that the only way to get my attention was to use my body as the beacon signalling me to come home to myself. I had so many opportunities to make changes, but I was too stubborn or stuck in my thoughts to heed the signs and move forward. I guess that's why I felt an urge to share my story: if only we could get out of our own way to allow real change to happen. Don't wait for the desperate moments where change is the only option. Look within now, do the work, and the rewards will be strikingly significant.

Could I really measure the changes in my life? Besides seeing small benefits from meditation, mindfulness, and the shedding of labels, could I really see and feel my viewpoint and outlook changing? Initially, maybe no. I still felt anger, could still raise my voice, could still feel slighted by a friend. But as I continued to work and be more open to receiving direction without trying to push it myself, I could see how—when I softened those hard edges—it felt good, better, lighter.

All these practices I put into place to ease my mind and racing thoughts as my body roller-coastered in ways both foreign and scary to me. I started the practices to bring myself under control and to find some peace in my otherwise tumultuous days. And they did do that. My meditation practice led to more mindfulness, which led to a greater level of gratitude. All three contributed to re-evaluating the labels I had patched onto myself and my relationship with the only person that mattered: me. While it all helped my body stay calm and grounded to heal, what was ultimately making the most difference was the way I was thinking.

So, after some time and facing many challenging situations, I could say that yes, I could see my viewpoint changing. The positive repetition I applied to my thoughts started to become a natural way of existing rather than a forced state, and I was starting to move through my day with a brighter outlook. When I was faced with challenges, I didn't hyperventilate and create worse-case scenarios. My natural go-to now was to acknowledge the situation, maybe have a moment of minute panic, but then look forward and ahead to moving through it. I was finding that issues from my past that would have had me reeling for days and months were now moments in life that, yes, needed to be dealt with but with a deep understanding that they didn't define me or my future. How I lived through those moments, learning and growing and surviving, was what defined me. How I breathed through the tough times—allowing myself to feel sadness, grief, and sorrow—was what gave me strength. I realized that feeling the emotions was warranted, but succumbing to fear and dropping my resolve were what would leave me powerless.

I know this because I lived it. I know this because it's true.

Chapter 25

THE WORRY HAS GOT TO GO

For my whole life I have been an emotional person. I didn't like to show affection or emotion outwardly, but inside I was a big ball of mush. I cried a lot when I was young, from heartbreak, disappointment, frustration, hurt. I felt things deeply and I often took on, unknowingly, the emotions or hurt of others. And as I said before, I was a worrier. I worried about everything. My parents often travelled together internationally for my dad's job and I always worried that something would happen to them. I was worried about my grades. I worried about what people thought of me. I was scared of the dark. But, most of all, I was worried about what would happen in the future.

Even through all this, I maintained being a glass-half-full person. I always felt that even when things seemed at their most terrible, tomorrow was another day and I could start anew. So I lived with a strange juxtaposition in my own self; optimism and hopefulness for the future, with worry and anxiousness about how I was going to get there.

While recovering, I realized that this absolutely needed to change. The worry was exhausting, and it permeated so much of my life that I knew it couldn't be healthy. That's where all the work really helped me and where I recognized the most growth and change. And I think that, on some level, worry or stress or anxiety is something that we all share, a common tenet that runs throughout most of our lives in some way. Of course, these emotions are needed and warranted to a degree because without them we likely might not get anything done. A slight anxiousness about a job interview, a mild stress about an upcoming test, whatever it may be, these emotions are natural and essential parts of our lives. They become troublesome when they penetrate more aspects of our lives than necessary and we can't outrun or overcome the incessant compounding of stress upon stress.

In our North American lifestyle, we place a lot of emphasis on getting things done, often multiple things at one time, racing against a clock that seems to tick faster and more urgently each day. I fell victim to this myself, especially when I placed unrealistic labels on myself for what equalled success and achievement. We want more, better, bigger, and often run ourselves ragged trying to get it. For some, they want to be better or have more than someone else. In others, it's a push to be better or bigger for a reason that can't ultimately be justified. While I wasn't someone who strived to achieve in order to outwit someone else, I did set high expectations for myself and tough deadlines to get there. As I continued to refocus my thoughts and approach situations in a different way, the more I realized that the pursuit of all these things at a rapid pace was futile. Worrying and stressing about the next job, the next phase, the next milestone was simply setting me and my health up for extra challenges that I certainly didn't need.

Let's put it this way: having goals and desires and hopes is what drives our lives. Being dreamers and setting high standards and goals for ourselves is an important way for our souls to grow and for each of us to reach our full potential. But it doesn't all have to be at the same time. I wanted it all at the same time. I had set goals for myself when I was in my early twenties that I hadn't come anywhere near achieving by the time I was in my forties. The goals weren't wrong; it was just my unrealistic expectation that I had to have it all, right now, in order to enjoy life.

When I stopped putting the stress on achieving something or being in a certain position at a specific time, things changed. I still had those goals, I still wanted to find meaningful work, help Andre to continue building his career, be mortgage- and debt-free, be healthy, have financial freedom... I still wanted and strived for all that. It's when I let go of the timeline that the changes started happening. The very things I constantly worried about just didn't seem to be that pressing anymore. I realized that if I took the time to sit back and evaluate what I wanted, how I was to get there became more clear.

I stopped worrying about how Sydney would develop and if she would make the right choices. I stopped worrying so intensely about our financial situation and whether we would ever be able to build savings. Most importantly, I stopped stressing and worrying about what was to become of me and where I would find my footing. An interesting thing happened when I let go and loosened my grip: things just happened. Sydney and I grew closer and I started to see her as the person she was, capable of handling herself and making good decisions for herself, not the person I worried she would become. Andre's business continued to build and it became interesting and challenging for him again. And I was allowing myself the time to be okay with where I was and not put the pressure on myself to have a job, or a firm direction. When I quieted down and allowed for the natural flow of life to happen, I began to find inspiration and joy in all the little things I did each day. I appreciated my role as Sydney's mom more. I enjoyed taking care of the home and the family more. I accepted that I was where I was supposed to be at that very moment. By moving more calmly and graciously through my daily life, I was allowing the right path to make itself known to me.

As I mentioned at the start of the book, I've always been fascinated with writing. I'm not a trained writer and I have never attempted to write anything of substance before. And in my attempt to "find" myself in those early years with Sydney, I didn't take the time to ask myself and really listen to where I wanted to be. I stressed and worried and panicked that I wasn't where I should be so I made decisions that I thought would easily get me there—ultimately leading me anywhere but up. All the starts and stops led me to this moment, to what I was going through, and I finally stopped the rollercoaster and stilled myself enough to feel what was next. I felt the inspiration to write it down not because I thought it would be my new direction but because I felt compelled to do so. And I didn't stress or worry about what the end result would be. I just let it flow and it felt great.

It felt like things were coming full circle and revealing their truth to me in every way. I worked hard initially to change the labels I'd put on myself for what equalled success and value. I spent time working through the fears and worries that served no purpose other than to add distress and ill health into my life. And here I was now, trying to let go of my control over things or my need to manipulate results in my favour. It all seemed to be interconnected: without one, the next couldn't be achieved. If I didn't see my value as being just me, I wouldn't have been able to relish and enjoy the everyday moments and simple occurrences that were springing up around me. When I dropped the label of what defined my worth, a career or a job; when I accepted that worry only closes the door to prosperity and abundance; and when I settled calmly and released control, my world got brighter. Not darker or smaller or more confining. It felt so much more open, rife with possibilities, there for the taking.

When I stopped running, it all stopped roller-coastering. For the first time in a really long time, things felt attainable. I had more hope in what life could be like, an underlying feeling that everything would be okay and that dreams, passions, and desires could actually become reality someday. It didn't have to be today, or next week, or before I was fifty. Lowering the benchmark of time allowed the idea to permeate more. Plus, the thought that success didn't have to be obtained at a young age in order to be enjoyed was liberating.

All these little things that popped up into focus now made the future seem even more attainable. How was it possible that by doing less, I felt I could achieve more? How could connecting with my family, enjoying my home, slowing down, and really settling in ignite the spark of possibility for doing it all? It was really an exciting place to be. Now that I had caught a glimpse, I didn't want to look back.

Chapter 26

IT'S OKAY TO BE HUMAN

It can seem altogether too simplistic and naive. Think good thoughts and your world will change. Talk nicely to yourself and your eyes will open. Think positively about what you want and you will manifest it into your reality. Whatever you think today will be your future. Blah, blah, blah. I'd heard and read it all before. And while I used to be fascinated by the idea of manifesting your own reality and I read books like The Secret and followed authors like Eckhart Tolle, I didn't really, actually believe that the concepts had any true merit or would actually produce the results I was hoping for, purely with belief and reliance on them alone. Plus, it looked time-consuming and difficult. I didn't have the time to create a vision board, or write in a journal, or list all my gratitude. In my heart I wanted to believe, I had glimmers of hope to believe, but my staunch thought that only hard work and sacrifice would get you there often won out.

My mistake early on was thinking that if I committed to envisioning my future, if I let go of trying to control the direction of my life, and if I allowed the flow of the Universe to guide me, then I would soon become someone I didn't recognize. Someone whose head was floating in the clouds on seeds of perceived hope rather than someone whose feet was firmly planted in the trenches, dealing with what was happening on the ground. How could I give warrant to the beautiful ideal of relinquishing fears and stepping fully into a life of Universal flow without looking and feeling like a lost soul who relies on chance rather than action? But my mistake was there. I had created the idea of a directionless, aimless person rather than one who stayed fully in control by allowing the abundance and direction to flow. The flow would happen regardless. By stepping in and following the stream, I wasn't giving up control but co-piloting my direction with much more determined purpose.

The fears, control issues, and stresses I had created only acted as barriers to the feelings of calm and joy that I ultimately craved. I could now see, through time and a relaxing of my held beliefs, that the less I struggled, the more I could achieve, both on a physical and material level and an emotional and spiritual level as well.

But all this didn't have to come at the expense of my human existence. I didn't have to stop feeling in order to see changes in my life. The assumption that I would be aimless was rooted in the idea that to let go and be free, so to speak, meant that I had to be void of any real emotion. Which would be near impossible for me: I'm an emotional person. I guess I had this vision of a carefree hippie person, living each moment to moment, day to day, without direction or concrete goals, but someone who was happy without stress. I had equated a stress-free, harmonious life with the Hollywood fodder of a laid-back slacker, which didn't really fit my ideals or persona. I didn't understand yet that that vision was all in my head, was one that I'd created. I could loosen the reins at any time and ride the energy of the Universal flow and still be me with feelings and emotions, goals and dreams.

This was important to remember. Throughout my entire healing process, I struggled with feelings of guilt when I would regress in my thought patterns. I would often chastise myself if I fell into old patterns and behaviours, admonishing myself for not moving forward emotionally. The lesson I needed to learn was that letting go of the old labels and fears and leaning into the flow didn't mean that I'd stop being human, stop feeling things. It was okay to cry if I needed to cry. It was okay to be angry if something upset me. Emotions were real and important and so very needed; the key, however, was to allow the emotion to simply be without attaching anything to it or without creating more of a story behind it.

After five years of recovery, I thought I'd finally turned a corner with my skin. Most of my body surface was new; I had grown new skin many times over and I could feel and see its firmness. But my face, neck, and chest remained a struggle. Even though I intuitively knew that recovery from topical steroid addition and the subsequent withdrawal followed a pattern, it was still difficult. I knew that my face would take longer to heal because it was the first place where topical steroid creams had been applied. The first location was always the last to heal. Even though I knew this and had witnessed the miracle of my body working, toiling, and living all on its own, I couldn't stop feeling the deep sadness when my face would continually cycle through ooze, extreme dryness, and sagging skin. I would see a little improvement and feel buoyed, only to find my skin flaring terribly just two days later. I remember feeling incredible one Sunday. We had booked a reservation at our favourite restaurant shortly after some lockdown restrictions were lifted. For the first time in about four months, I was able to see some significant improvement in the skin on my face. I was excited about going out after a long hiatus and took a lot of time in the bathroom doing my hair and applying my makeup. It felt great to look at myself and feel like a bit of me was back. I hadn't been able to wear any makeup for much of the previous year so for someone like me, who loved playing around with and wearing makeup every day, this particular Sunday was a real treat.

And I looked great, felt great. We had a wonderful meal and the good feeling lasted into the evening and the next morning. This was the turning point: I was back. Clearer sailing from here.

By Tuesday, my face had declined significantly. My eyelids and surrounding skin were oozing and the pulling and tightness in my skin around my jawline made it difficult to open my mouth to eat. I went into a tailspin. I held myself together enough to see Sydney off to school and Andre off to work and then I just gave in. I was so traumatized that I transported back to the early days, when I was desperate and depressed. I cried, hard angry tears and gulping sobs. I cursed God, I lashed out, and I screamed. I'd been working so hard on all aspects of my life and now, after five years of recovering, I was plunged back into a flare that felt so demoralizing I didn't know how I could go on.

But then the tears subsided. As I hiccupped my way back to calm, I felt the release of my anger and fear. I realized one important message from that experience. I had been working on "fixing" myself so I could traverse through my life in joy and loving each moment, seeing the light in every activity and the grandeur of all that was around me. My quest for physical healing and connecting more fully to my spirit meant, at least in my mind, that those tough moments wouldn't get me down anymore, they wouldn't affect me in the same way they used to. I'd been working toward ultimate contentment, and when I had my physical setback and I raged, I was initially so disappointed in myself. Had I not been changing my viewpoint and releasing my fears and unhealthy labels so that I could navigate through my life and *not* fall off the rails? Wasn't my whole goal now to be calmer and ride the wave?

But that's what this new flare opened my eyes to see. Above all else, I am still human, with feelings and emotions and hurts. I could rewire myself through a more positive lens, but that didn't mean I needed to be numb to what was going on around me. Being angry and upset was okay—necessary, actually. What was important to remember about changing my perspective was how I reacted after I reacted. It was about allowing the moments to happen but then let them pass, without judgment, without holding on.

And that's what happened. I was angry and sad and moped around for a couple of days, but I didn't fight the emotions, nor did I give them more weight than they deserved. I didn't allow the fear-mongering to happen, I didn't allow my thoughts to be transformed into a future fear of laboured recovery. I didn't let my thoughts run wild about possible negative outcomes or how much time it would take to heal from this latest flare. I lived in the moment, at the moment.

I guess that was the real lesson: to live in the moment, at the very time it is happening. To allow yourself to feel, whether sadness or light, defeated or elated. To live and feel right at that time and allow the flow without pretence of what else may come. To engage with whatever you are faced with and deal with it in the moment. The next hour, the next day was a new moment. Perhaps that was the magic that had eluded me before. The calm I desired, the status quo, the peace, wasn't found in erasing hardship, or finally just getting through something. It was found in being present in whatever the moment gave me and moving through it in real time, without projections into the future. The peace was found in knowing that this one moment doesn't define the rest of the moments. It challenges me and possibly pushes me to my limits, but it builds a resiliency to weather any storm. To live a life that is not wrapped up in future predictions. To live a life in which I feel deeply in exactly where I am at that moment.

It was okay to be sad if my health took two steps back. It was, and is, okay to work hard on changing things in your life and then somedays feel like it's not worth it. It's okay to not know if you can endure and go on.

This is life and reality and not something that is embarrassing. As we push ourselves to be better people—not for others but for ourselves—we will be faced with obstacles and presented with triumphs, even when we think we're pulling through and nearing an end. The triumphs are easy to celebrate, but we must also learn to appreciate the obstacles. The real gift is realizing that it's okay to feel, but that the emotion and the uncertainty exist in just one moment in time: a small moment in the otherwise vast timeline of life. All the hard work—the changing of thought patterns, releasing of labels, demolishing of outside expectations, all of it—is and will always be worth it. It will always be what fills most of life's moments, and ultimately it is what forms the fabric of life each day so that setbacks are mere bumps that soon become pebbles.

Chapter 27

PATIENCE IS A VIRTUE THAT HEALS

So much of what I was learning seemed to be common sense: to love myself, to speak to myself kindly, to operate from love. How simple it all was to say, yet so difficult to actually do. The truth, I was discovering, was that no one else stood in the way of me doing those things. My fate and my reality were not machinations of the world around me or of my relationships or of my family. They were entirely in my palm, and the stories I told myself were the walls I'd built up around me to prevent the good stuff from reaching me.

By now I had initiated mindfulness and gratitude into my daily practice, resulting in a natural shift in my focus to see the positive first. I noticed small improvements in how I thought about myself and my place in the world. Slowing down, calming the mind, and rewiring my thought patterns had kicked into gear significant changes that could be maintained for good. But the most valuable lesson that I was learning was to be patient.

It's not that the "me before" was an impatient person. I wasn't impulsive, preferring to weigh all my options and think them through. But I did like things to move along. I liked to see action and was ready to be on to the next thing. I wanted resolutions, and my impatience usually reared up when things just dragged on.

I knew when I started my journey of not using topical steroid creams that I would have to face waiting and would need to sharpen my patience skills. As with many things, though, what we anticipate and prepare for is rarely enough for the actual event. I didn't think I would have to find as much patience as I actually ended up needing. My healing took place at such a snail's pace, I would feel immense frustration at not seeing results quicker. Especially in the earlier years, when everything was still new to me, it was difficult to watch such slow improvement. The body, though, does not have a timeline, and I had to succumb to the mercy of something I had no control over.

That's where the lesson of patience comes in. It's not an easy one to master, though. Waiting sometimes seems futile, and I was left many times feeling like I was wasting time, that I should be and could be doing more. I even felt like life was passing me by. We live in a society that values accomplishment and we like to tick things off our living agenda, so when that wasn't possible for me, it felt like everyone else was forging ahead, making those accomplishments, reaching those milestones, ticking more off their lists than I could ever manage to do. Having patience in our fast-forward, perpetually moving world is a virtue that often just doesn't seem possible

Or does it?

I was forced to have patience during my physical recovery because there were no remedies, cures, or support that I could tap into to push my healing forward. Only time could do that, and I needed to dig deep to find a well of patience since everything was literally out of my control. I started to wonder, though, that if I was more patient in other areas of my life, would it feel less hectic and frantic? If I just allowed the Universe to unfold its treasures at its own pace, would I be more receptive to the little miracles that can happen every day?

I'll admit that if I hadn't been knocked down by my physical limitations during my topical steroid withdrawal, I may not have committed to slowing down and being more patient. Sure, I believed I had enough patience for the things that really mattered: parenting Sydney, dealing with financial obstacles, working on our family. But the kind of patience that I'm talking about now is the type that asks us to stop and breathe. To close our eyes for a moment and appreciate where we are. I was so anxious to get on with things, with my life, that I didn't have the patience to sit and wait. I am forever grateful for the time I was forced to sit and wait, even though it was fraught with discomfort, as it awarded me with the feeling of just how empowering it is to have patience with life and patience with my direction in it.

This is not a passive exercise, though. Having patience with how life will unfold doesn't mean to give over control to the Universal force. Life still needs a driver, and we are at the wheel of our very own journeys. Goals, plans, and dreams are integral parts of a soul's journey, and I knew that giving up and allowing some other force to take over was not the lesson to learn. Rather, setting my intentions and then cultivating a practice of patience to allow the Universe to carry those intentions was what I needed to master. As I sat patiently waiting for my body to physically heal, I was rewarded with improvements, even small ones, that reinforced my belief in the power of our own selves.

Instead of pushing and controlling how I thought I wanted my life to develop, I allowed the space and time for things to manifest without my direct intention. I still dreamed of what I hoped my life would look like once I healed and I still set goals for where I wanted to be. But I calmed down and settled, allowing the intention to marinate while staying open to what the result would be. Ultimately, this patience allowed me to inquire deeper into my soul about what I really wanted to do and where I really wanted to go, without the limitations of specific timelines for completion or a designated roadmap of how to get there. With patience, I soon realized that I would start to allow more options and more outcomes to be expressed simply by waiting for them to be.

In the patient moments, I listened to my heart and my intuition to write things down and allowed myself the time to write—something I had been aching to do. I didn't have an intention of where it would lead me, but I knew if I kept patient, the right outcome would happen. I also found the time to help Andre transition his business and start fresh.

Having the patience to know that—through intention, dedication, and hard work—we could build his business again and see results that could far outreach our expectations. By freeing myself from the deadlines and timelines and the personal demands for firm completion and definitive outcomes, I allowed the energy to flow in a more harmonious way. And if it didn't happen today, I knew it would happen tomorrow, or the next day. I just had to have the patience to wait for the goodness to come.

Chapter 28

FIND IT WITHIN

By the time I was writing my second or third draft of this book, it had been close to six years since I'd last used steroid creams for my eczema. I had been in recovery for more than 2,100 days. My daughter had gone from a middle-school student to an adolescent in high school. It had been more than half a decade. More than half a decade.

Part of me was dumbfounded and angry that I, like so many thousands around the world, had been prescribed something that would steal more than five years of my life simply because I chose not to use it again. And while I still lived and made memories and laughed during those years, the dark cloud of repeated flares and a debilitating physical presence definitely made that time much less joyful than it could have and should have been. For that alone, I will continue to be an advocate for reform in the dermatological community regarding its approach to alleviate and cure skin conditions. For that alone, I will, without hesitation, scream from the rooftops, "Never use any topical steroid treatment for eczema ever." Period.

I can't deny, however, that if it weren't for that initial push to stop the steroid creams, I may not be in the position I'm in now. Had life just continued along and I hadn't made the connection with the overuse of these creams to my various health issues, I would probably still be stuck in my worrying mind frame and the constant stress of what was next. Sometimes I was angry with myself for not taking better care of the whole me earlier, that I had to be in a health crisis and literally housebound to take the time to go deeper and work to heal my spirit. Maybe it would have made recovery easier and shorter if I'd already begun that work. Then I realized that it wasn't *until* I went through my struggle with topical steroid withdrawal that I was ready to accept the challenge to work on myself fully and commit to the practice of rewiring my thoughts and changing my outlook. I wouldn't have been able to do one without the other.

That doesn't mean, though, that there needs to be a significant health or life crisis to push us to make changes in our lives. I just wasn't tuned in enough to get there before, but our bodies and the world around us are always giving us signs and opportunities to change for the better. The key is to be aware and open to the messages when they arrive.

It's hard to make changes. Deep down we often know we need to, but we just can't seem to get there. We know work is making us stressed, we know we need to spend more time with our kids, we know that some of our choices are unhealthy and unproductive. Yet even though we know all this, the fear of change and disruption traps us from making any significant headway in our behaviours and thoughts.

Some things in life are unavoidable. Particular limitations may mean that we can't change our jobs and so work-related stress may always be present. But nurturing ourselves and treating our bodies and minds with kindness and love can help combat the other circumstances that we can't control at the moment. I certainly didn't look at ways to be more selfish and cradle myself when the fear took a tight hold of my emotions and thoughts. I didn't give voice to the fact that while something in my life may not be going the exact way I had hoped, I could control so much more and it starts with my own relationship to myself. Talking kindly to myself, viewing myself with a softer lens, and finding activities and situations that help to nourish my soul were and are ways to shift the focus from fear and stress to love, acceptance, and joy.

When I was going through my withdrawal, I was never in a place that I wanted to be in. The unpredictability of when a flare may appear and its severity made maintaining and building my event planning business almost impossible. I wasn't able to confidently know how I would be feeling physically, so booking client meetings, conducting on-site visits, and even participating in industry trade shows were impossible. The business I wanted to grow just fizzled. I also didn't feel confident enough to embark in any new direction. Retraining myself, attending lectures, or delving into a different career all had to sit on the back burner while I succumbed to the whims of my body and its healing journey. I was definitely not where I wanted to be. But even among that stress and the fear of not knowing where I was headed or when I would get there, when I breathed deeply and reminded myself that as with everything else this too will have an end, I was able to compartmentalize the ideas of where I should be (the ego's list of where I should be at a certain point in my life) and where I actually was (where my spirit was, right here in the moment) into separate entities of my existence. The stress and fear of not knowing were real, but only as real as I was willing to give life to them. I absolutely could not change my physical journey; I was where I was and no amount of worry or stress could or would push my journey along any faster. So softening my lens and looking at myself with more kindness ultimately abated the fear, worry, and stress, allowing me to live not necessarily in a place I had envisioned or intended at the moment but maybe someplace better and more real. When some circumstances are out of our control, in turning toward ourselves and embracing the relationship with our thoughts, emotions, and physicality, we can find more strength, courage, and love than we ever thought possible. And with that strength, courage, and love comes an understanding that the only thing that matters is the joy we create in our spirits and in our hearts. Everything else is just an illusion that ebbs and flows and changes and moves. The true reality, and all that truly is, is found within ourselves.

Chapter 29

COULD FORGIVENESS BE THE KEY?

Reviewing all the ideas and concepts that had opened my thinking revealed one universal truth. That all of this—all the joy, acceptance, love, and life in all its entirety—held one tenet at its core: forgiveness.

A lot of my worries and anxieties were rooted in some form of animosity or hurt from someone else. It was from friends who wronged me, or the opportunity that someone else grabbed, and even some people who left our friendship without a discussion or closure.

To move forward, though, to really live in this moment and embrace all the wonders and joy available at any given time, I had to let go, to breath and to forgive. With my relationships that fizzled out during my healing, I had to forgive the other person for the energy they took from me, and I had to forgive myself for not closing that chapter sooner. I needed to let go of the animosity, both real and perceived, to allow space for the good parts of life to filter more readily. Forgiving someone else or a situation in which we don't feel we have control over is a necessary and important step in releasing and moving forward in a more prosperous way. It is easier said than done in many situations, but it is so very important to our soul's growth and for us to achieve an even more enhanced quality of life.

Even without forgiveness, life still moves on. In fact, we can live quite happily and productively without honouring forgiveness by just simply carrying on. Continuing to harbour resentment or hold on to past hurts doesn't affect our daily living, so for all intents and purposes, real forgiveness doesn't seem to improve much on the surface of things. So it's easy to say that we forgive and move on without realizing that we haven't let go of the thought and emotion attached to the feeling. Of course, I could *say* that I had moved on when a situation or person had wronged me, but many times I didn't *actually* move on in my thoughts. I would go back, revisit, replay, get hurt again, feel angry again, move on. Repeat, repeat, repeat.

By continuing to unintentionally hold on to past angers or resentments, I was constricting my body into a vice of tension, resulting over time in physical pain, emotional strain, and fervent thoughts of negativity. I wanted to feel lighter and more free, and forgiveness is the only way to reach that level of detachment.

Actual, real forgiveness is found in the acceptance of the situation that is at hand and of the shifting perspective and thoughts about it as a whole. I needed to realize that no amount of anger or resentment that I held could ever change what the outcome was. No matter how much I held on to the idea that I was wronged, it wouldn't change what had occurred in the past, and no amount of berating myself for situations I didn't control better could ever alter the outcome of today. It just wouldn't. The past was in the past, where it needed to stay, not propelled into the present and future by my invisible horseman. The thought wave and energy I projected today needed to be free of the vibrations of yesterday.

It's an interesting perspective. The reality that no matter how much we want them to, our thoughts today will never change the past. Ever. But what today's thoughts will do is shape what happens to us in the future—and that is a guarantee. Holding on to hurts and resentments doesn't serve any purpose; in fact, it only sets us up for more of the same disappointments and aggravation in the future.

So forgiving someone else is imperative for our spirit's growth and prosperity here on Earth. But even more important to our soul is the ultimate act of kindness: forgiveness of ourselves.

I am a fairly optimistic person, and throughout my life I have tried to look on the positive side of many situations. I know that a lot of my friends who have faced setbacks and trials do very much the same: deal with it and move on. Keep moving forward. I think that's a great quality to nurture and foster a sense of tenacity. The piece I didn't pay much attention to was the negative talk I gave to myself.

Much of my worry and stress was in some form of disappointment or concern with myself. A disappointment in how I handled a situation, in not thinking of myself first, or even in allowing myself to be in certain situations. When I examined my thoughts and feelings, it usually involved some aspect of thinking of the past and reliving a moment in which I should have acted differently or taken a different course. Even when other people were concerned, I realized that I would often go back in time and admonish myself for not seeing the signs sooner or for allowing myself to share my life or parts of myself with another who didn't deserve that opportunity. I found that I lived a lot in regret.

Mixed in with all my fun memories and accomplishments, my story included much too much negative spin, with the finger usually pointing in my direction.

If forgiveness of others is important, then forgiveness of ourselves is crucial. By forgiving ourselves for any part that we may have played in past hurts or actions that allowed us to carry resentments through, we release the angst and turmoil that blocks the passage of true, unfiltered good. But how do we really forgive ourselves? It's simple: we just do. By looking at ourselves with the kindness and tenderness that we would show a child learning how to navigate through life, we cradle ourselves in warm love that doesn't ask for or need validation and reconciliation from anyone else. When we forgive ourselves we actually validate ourselves. We acknowledge to the Universe that we are valuable, important, and worthy. We accept that our position in this world at this time is right and that our contributions and existence are worth something. If we can offer the gift of forgiveness to someone else then we must allow that same gift to be received by ourselves as well.

Chapter 30

SO MUCH TO LEARN

My whole life underwent a major transformation at a time when I wasn't searching for it—or even wanting it, to be honest. Life threw some things at me and after muddling through and dragging my feet to seek out some answers, I took it upon myself to find a way to heal my body and finally be free from the constraints of chronic eczema. Like most things we endeavour to do, what I ended up getting was not what I had envisioned.

In the end, it was so much more. I found a new and heightened appreciation of what I have and of all the beauty that surrounds me each day. It was through the darkest of times that I was able to see what a gift each new day is, where I felt an immense appreciation for the little things like walking, exercising, laughing, family. While I always felt grateful for all the things in my life, I realized that I didn't give them the full value that they deserved. I took things for granted, like they would always be there. I saw first-hand how that just isn't true. Our life can change in unintended and often difficult ways. Without being able to recognize the good, we can spiral.

I also found a deeper connection spiritually. I was able to see how everything was interrelated to each other and how we are all spiritual, soulful people, looking for purpose and meaning in our life's journey. I was shown that while our bodies are our vessels with which to traverse this world, they are not who we are at our very essence. Who we are doesn't change when our outside changes. Our desires, hopes, dreams, ambitions, talents, and interests remain, even when we may not be physically able to achieve them. I needed to reconnect to who I was in order to do what I wanted.

Influence from outside sources doesn't have a place in our journey here. What someone else thinks we should be doing, or the judgments that others put on us, have no bearing on the trajectory that our lives can take and of all that we can achieve. Most importantly, the conversations that we have with ourselves, the truths we allow ourselves to acknowledge, weigh far greater on our happiness and success than any other outside recognition ever could.

I realized how valuable our health really is. How the saying "health is the real wealth" has never been more poignant or true. Without our health, we have nothing. I had to learn that lesson the hard way, but I am ever so grateful that I was given the opportunity to do so. If I had not been open to the lessons and learning at the time they were presented to me, I may have gone through another twenty years of my life not grasping all that was available to me.

My most important realization is that gratitude and being grateful for all that I have is the key to abundance in all that I want. It took a lot of time for me to come to that conclusion and to make the necessary changes in myself to operate from a grateful heart in all that I do. It wasn't easy. A lifetime of anxiety, worry, and stress was a difficult cloak to shed. Those thoughts still try to creep in, but my confidence and resolve remind me to banish those thoughts and to focus on gratitude. Whenever I feel overwhelmed—whether it be from bills, house payments, personal relationships, whatever—I stop, turn inward, and remind myself that all of that is just an illusion. It is only real to the degree of thought that I give to it. Life will carry on no matter what I think or feel. Those financial commitments or difficult situations will never leave when I worry or stress, and it is best to forge forward with an attitude of faith and hope, knowing that the Universe has my back.

As far as my health was concerned, I will admit that it was extremely difficult to find gratitude or positivity when I was in the midst of the most physically debilitating times. As anyone with any chronic condition or who has experienced any kind of ceaseless pain will tell you, gratefulness is the furthest thing from your mind. In the absence of health, what could I possibly be grateful for?

That was my biggest mental challenge. I found a definite resolve when I worked through all my mental roadblocks and challenged myself to align with more purpose to my desires and wants in life. I felt a sense of calm when I shed the labels and focused on my direction without thought or concern over what others thought or what was expected of me. And through all the years, it was working. I was moving through recovery feeling like I was going to be a better person on the other side. In the good times physically, when there were days, months even, of reprieve, this resolve held steady. But as my physical recovery had its many ebbs and flows, ups and downs, so too did my feeling of gratitude about where I was.

I knew that I was extremely lucky, regardless of where my health was at the time. I knew in my heart that I had been blessed with so many wonderful experiences and my life was rich and full. In the hard times, though, no amount of grateful remembering could soften my feelings of life letting me down. I could say my prayers and recite all the things I was grateful for, but I didn't really *feel* it at times; like I was just going through the motions because this was now my new routine. I didn't feel grateful sometimes; I felt angry, let down, hopeless. I had many dark moments to navigate.

Over time, I kept getting through it, and on the other side of the pain and hopelessness, I saw the miracle of tenacity and how unpredictable life can be, even in the good things. Just as quickly as life can be difficult, it can shift into calm and wonderful. And when looking at things from a calm perspective, I realized that I always have something to be grateful for.

This practice has absolutely changed my life in ways that are sometimes difficult to articulate. Before, I gave thanks for the things I had, wrote in a gratitude journal, and basically went through the motions of what I had read and thought I should be doing. I worked on changing my thoughts to change my perspective, and I performed the daily rituals with the same perfunctory approach as I would a to-do list. I did what I needed to do, but I didn't feel what I needed to feel. As I lived more with the physical limitations at times and subsequent healing that followed, I saw how merely performing actions wasn't enough to find the true and lasting change in myself. I needed to feel it, to become it, to live it. The easiest and most profound way for me to do that was to start and end each day from a position of gratitude.

When I saw my body heal, I was amazed at how resilient and remarkable our bodies are and how often I took for granted what I would do each day. I never gave a thought to being able to walk from my car to the grocery store, or to run up a flight of stairs. Taking a shower or using my hands to cut flowers were normal, everyday actions that never occupied much, if any, of my thoughts. Now, though, I saw everything through a different lens. How lucky I was that I could go for a walk. How wonderful was it to be able to luxuriate in a hot shower. And how rich was the nature surrounding me. I began to see the greatness in all the things I encountered and, quite frankly, my luck at being a part of it.

A strange thing began to happen. As I made the effort to appreciate my life, from a simple moment like sitting down for a great cup of tea to the more profound experience of being able to pay all my bills on time, the beauty of everything became more obvious. As I practised a true gratitude more, more things appeared to be grateful for. In the beginning, I tried to remember not to take anything for granted and to consistently practise gratitude. But as time progressed, I soon found that I didn't need to look for things to be grateful for, I was just grateful. Grateful for the new day, grateful for a beautiful view, grateful for my health, grateful for changing nature.

This view through gratitude also aligned wonderfully with the work I had done to release the labels and expectations I had carried with me for far too long. With gratitude I didn't feel any pressure or desire to compare myself to anyone else. I didn't need to gauge my success against another, or use any internal metric to calculate my worth. I was grateful for me and I was grateful for everyone else. It was that simple.

So now, I start each day giving thanks for being here. Giving thanks that I allowed my body to heal. Giving thanks that I pushed my insecurities, fears, anxieties, and stresses away to allow for all the beauty of the world to shine through. Grateful that I was given the opportunity to right my path and embrace everything that's given to me: all the challenges, hardships, joy, and celebrations. Grateful that as crazy and messy and hurtful as life can get, it is also beautiful and exciting and full of joy. It is our choice how we wish to view it.

Chapter 31

IT'S A PLACE OF JOY

It's a rainy slow day today, but as I sip my tea and gaze out my window, I feel grateful to be in the place where I am. I never would have anticipated that day in January more than six years ago that I would be where I am right at this moment. My five-year plan had greater aspirations for my life, both professionally and physically. I had imagined that my event planning business would have grown, that I would have stretched into other exciting areas professionally, and that at forty-five I would have a good idea of where I was going and what the road ahead looked like.

I am nowhere near where I had imagined.

In some respects, if I hadn't decided to stop using all steroid creams and plunge myself into withdrawal, I likely would have achieved all that I had set out to do. I probably would have worked hard on building a brand, supporting Andre's business, and helping Sydney navigate adolescence.

Life would have easily bumped along, and quite possibly I could have been exactly where I find myself now.

On the other hand, it may not have. Equally as possible, my limiting beliefs and anxieties easily could have hampered my growth professionally and I may not have been any further ahead. I could still be spinning my wheels, pushing an agenda that placed value only on work and professional achievements. The truth is, I just don't know.

What I do know is that I did make that decision to stop using steroid creams, and I am where I am now because of it. In a place of much more peace. In a place of much more acceptance. In a place of much more gratitude. I can see now what a gift it has been to be able to break down my internal barriers and learn to live in a place that is right only for me, without apologies or conditions. I am in a place that tells me that no comparison to others will ever satisfy my soul. I am in a place that allows me to see the joy around me without worry of what comes next. I am in a place that listens only to the voice and knowing in my heart of what I want and where I want to be.

The urgency for success that I once felt no longer plagues me. I have removed the timelines that I set out for myself in order to measure my worth and value. I now allow myself to live in a Universe that supports me and has my back if I just allow what is to be, to be. I haven't given up my dreams, or my aspirations. I am not idly sitting by and waiting for the Universe to make it happen for me. But I am relaxing into the energy and flow of a life that will unfold as it may. The grips of fear and worry have almost disappeared, replaced by a knowledge that, if I allow it, life will unfold in wonderful ways. There will always be challenges and setbacks, triumphs and joy—there always was. Now, though, I have stopped trying to manipulate and control how it all unfolds and am learning to live in an energetic flow. I experience the world now not by what I haven't achieved but in the so many ways that I can have, do, and experience more.

I have said a few times throughout this writing that my journey was divinely orchestrated. I believe that more than ever. Whatever push sent me on this journey was not one that originated organically from me alone. There was a knowing, a gnawing to step into something unknown and heal. I had been given this choice before, but for whatever reason I wasn't in the right mind space to accept the invitation. Now, my spirit knew I was capable of handling the challenge and that I would receive the gift of full healing if I was ready to allow it in.

My approach to life now is not dissimilar to how I was living before. I am still as optimistic as I always was, I still crave learning, I still strive to improve in any way that I can. These core values that define who I am are not lost in my new perspective. But where I was skeptical and hesitant before, I am now a believer. I believe in my own purpose, I believe in the power of the Universe, and I believe in our inherent right to feel love and joy in everything we encounter. And I realize too that everything I want and need and desire is within my reach. And while we all must participate in our lives in ways that continue to drive it forward, participating with an emotional and mental effort is just as important as participating with a physical one. Our minds play a much larger role in what life can offer us, and it is often the very act of engaging and enhancing our mental game that can help us see real positivity in our lives.

When I speak to myself now, it is with love and awe. It is with an understanding and an amazement of where I am in this wonderful world and where I can head. When I give gratitude now, I don't just say it, I feel it, deeply. Even the smallest of things I am grateful for, and I take time to activate the emotion in my heart and in my mind. This makes the experience so much richer. When I have doubt or fear now, I can lovingly push it aside, knowing that it is my positive intentions that will help steer my life in the direction I want, and that negative thoughts only push my desires further away from me.

I have been given the gift of insight and revelation, of truth and reality. I have been shown that we are wonderful, complicated, and beautiful people. I have been privileged to have a front-row seat for the wonders and intricacies of our world, Universe, and existence. And I can say with total clarity and conviction that life is worth living.

But the living must come from within us, from a desire and need to fulfill our soul's path. The simplest way to get there is to just be quiet and listen to ourselves. Our heart will tell us, our soul will guide us.

I have learned that the stories we tell ourselves are the best way to throw us off course. That the lies we perpetuate only serve one purpose: to diminish our glow. Our success, our path, and our ultimate joy is found in embracing who we are and emanating that out to the world. We must champion ourselves, we must believe in only ourselves.

I thought that I was my own cheerleader and advocate throughout my life. And I was, and continue to be. But I wasn't aware of the damage that my negative thoughts, feelings, and emotions were having on my ultimate pursuit of sustained happiness and joy. I was asleep to the key component to my health and well-being, and I didn't realize the extent to which I was playing the main role in suppressing my true joy. I am awake now and ready to move forward in love and happiness, forgiveness and joy.

I also now know that we must be accountable to ourselves. We must go deep, pushing against our held beliefs and detrimental thoughts to find a kinder, gentler place from which to operate. It isn't easy work, and it isn't work that can be done by someone else. Humbling ourselves to accept our faults, make decided efforts to overcome that which stalls us, and commit to continually working on our mental and spiritual health will lead us to a life that is brighter, warmer, and kinder. I am just like you, and you like me. We are all here to experience life and joy and, yes, love. We all, at our core, want to have many of the same things but most important is happiness and freedom. Freedom to feel good, freedom from our thoughts, freedom to create, and freedom to be who we truly are. But no one is like anyone else. While we all crave and thrive for many of the same things, there is only one of each of us. And while it may seem overplayed and oversaid, the uniqueness of each of us is needed and warranted and desired here, right now. We are all the same, yet no one is like another.

There is no magic needed to create the perfect life. There is no miracle that saves us from disease and misfortune. We have no way of knowing what our future holds for us, but we have the power within ourselves to help shape it and curate it through our thoughts, emotions, and desires. By building a strong relationship between tenacity and hard work, optimism and gratitude, we can open the doors to an abundance that is waiting for us all. An abundance that is ours to savour, to appreciate and to delight in. One that is unique to only us. Inside us is the key, and it is our job to turn it open.

Acknowledgements

There are many people along my journey of life so far that have influenced me in so many ways. While each interaction, each moment has woven a fabric of experiences in which I draw on for motivation and inspiration, there are some that have entered my life that have profoundly affected me, my life and my journey through this book. I have to give many thanks to my freelance editor Heather Sangster for being kind to this first time author and staying true to my original voice. Your edits and suggestions helped to bring better shape to the book and I am lucky to have you on my team. I give big hugs to my life-long friends, Stacey, Shannon and Maha. You have all seen me at my worst and been there for the best. Thank you for the times I leaned on you and you held me without judgement. I look forward to many, many more years of sharing life together. Thank you to my soul sisters Heather and Margarett. You both helped me to not only connect to my celestial team, but to my own inner spirit, helping to guide me along to my true path. You listened, you advised and I am so grateful to have met you both. There are four very special people in my life who have been by my side every step of the way, providing guidance and encouragement, comfort and love. I without a doubt, could not have taken this step without my mom Vicki, my dad Ralph, my husband Andre and my daughter Sydney. Through everything and always they are my rocks and my foundations. My dad's spirit had transcended before this book came fully together, but I know that he was and is always with me. His unwavering support in everything I did instilled a sense of hope and optimism in me regardless of circumstance. His sense of confidence is something I try to aspire to, and he lives forever in my heart. My mom was my first reader of the final manuscript and it was her opinion that mattered the most to me. If my mom liked it, then I knew it was okay. She is my confidant and someone I rely on for almost everything. I would not be where I am or who I am without her unwavering support, encouragement and love. I can't express enough the luck that was given to me when I met Andre, and I could never have known the trials and tribulations, elations and joys we would experience together. And even though I had hoped that we could weather any storm together, it wasn't until my withdrawal journey that I was shown the true capacity of love and the lengths that someone would go to support their partner. I feel blessed to have him with me as we traverse this life together. Sydney is the joy that I didn't know I needed. She has filled my soul with so much light that I often feel like my heart might just burst into a thousand pieces. She teaches me everyday how to lead with kindness and her positivity and go-getter attitude is something that I try to emulate each moment of the day. I am forever grateful to the Universe for trusting her to me. And I am most grateful and thankful to have taken this journey, to have been prompted and nudged by divine intervention to trust in myself to heal and to share my story with you.

About the Author

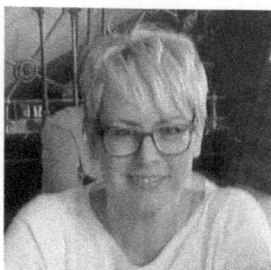

Allyson Steedman is a former corporate event planner and entrepreneur. Her many endeavours include owning a specialty dog boutique, a party planning and consulting business and a bespoke travel company. Her first hand experience with physical healing and emotional discovery has set her on a path to help others reignite their connection to their own spirit to help find joy, passion and abundance in their own lives. An avid learner, she is usually found nose deep in a book, playing her piano, and exploring the world. She lives in the suburbs of Toronto with her husband, daughter and dog.